THRESHOLDS

connecting body and soul
after brain injury

THRESHOLDS

connecting body and soul
after brain injury

by: lawrence m. pray with david gumm

RUDER FINN PRESS

"Surely God is in this place and I did not know it."

Genesis 28:16

table of contents

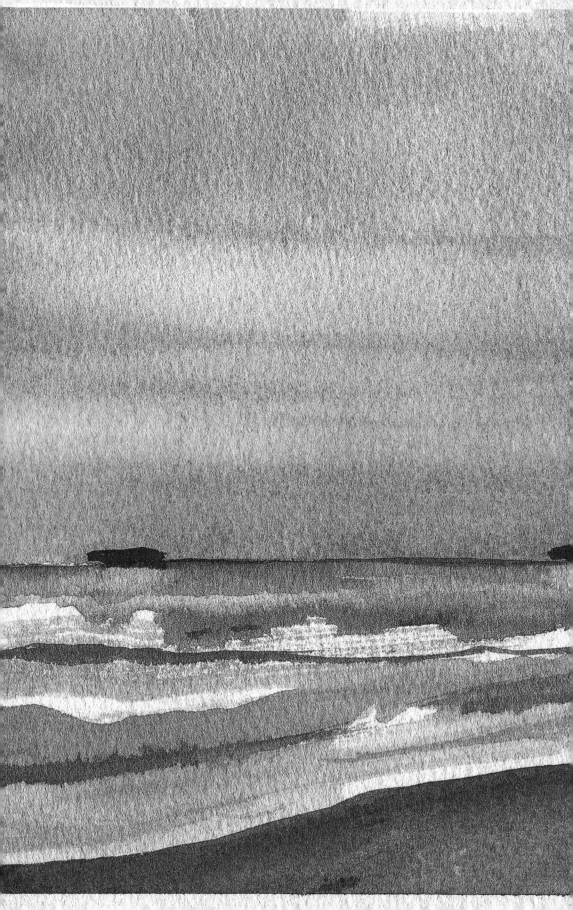

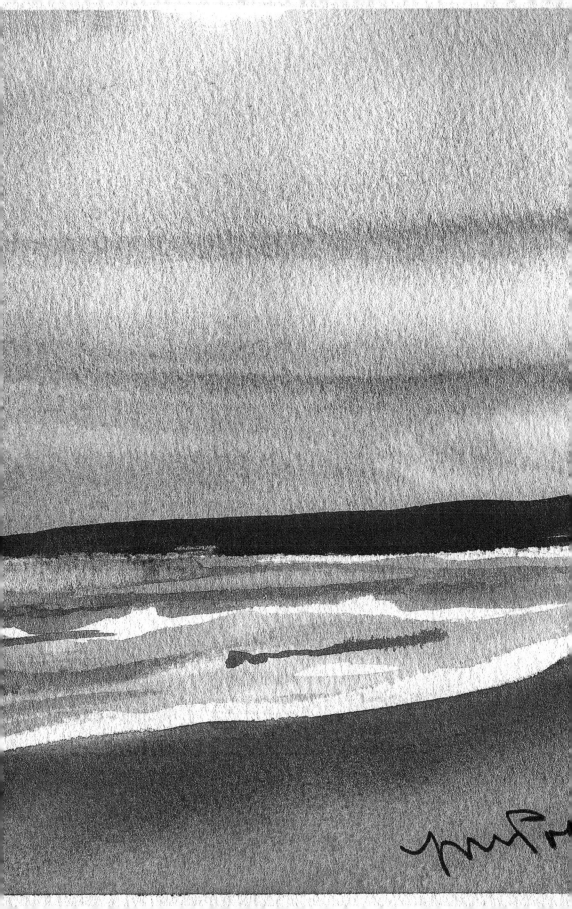

introduction

...

It is rarely good news when a pastor's phone rings after midnight. And so it was when Helen called.

"Larry," she said. "Floyd's had a stroke."

"Oh no," I said.

"The ambulance is on its way."

"I'll be right there." I rushed over and arrived just as the EMTs wheeled him from their house to the ambulance for a trip to the Emergency Room. One moment he had been full of life. A moment later he had fallen to the floor and could scarcely speak or move. The doctors did what they could and quickly admitted him to the hospital. A few days later they transferred him to the nursing home wing reserved for those needing acute care.

Over the next few weeks we did what churches and pastors do when life takes a turn for the worse. We encouraged each other, we held out for hope, listened three times over to every word the doctor said, and joined together in prayer. We kept in check our unspoken fear: Floyd might not make it. The man before us was a different person from the one we had known. His eyes carried messages words could not find. When I visited him over the next few days, he was often resting from some invisible activity that sapped his strength. Simply summoning strength to move from one moment to the next exhausted him.

One afternoon I stopped by, wondering again how to best connect with him when his speech was uncertain and sporadic at best. I greeted him with a "Glad to see you" smile and spoke a few words. He nodded and struggled to say a word or two. It was then my turn to nod as words escaped us both. I wasn't sure what he could understand and whether or not speech could establish a heartfelt conversation. Together we were bewildered. His eyes surveyed a strange landscape in which thought no longer freely connected to speech, in which perception itself was somehow unconnected to all he had once known. I sensed his thoughts circling and searching for words to convey a glimpse of this new experience. I had entered his room knowing we would pray, and he saw me knowing the same thing. There was no such thing as a pastoral visit without prayer. But story precedes prayer. There is a rhythm to pastoral ministry. Make the visit, gather the story, find the need, and offer a prayer that conveys both. Before we could pray I had to ask a question he might or might not be able to answer.

"What's it like, Floyd?" I asked, reaching out for his hands. "What's a stroke like?" He caught the question and let it sink in.

"Well," he said carefully, "it's not like I thought it would be." Like almost all of us, he knew people who suffered a stroke or two, and wondered what the sudden change was like.

With that, our conversation ended and prayer began. We gave thanks that he had survived, thanks for the doctors, and thanks for the nursing home. We asked for the strength to heal, for patience to understand what happened and for courage to keep fear at bay. Several weeks later, Floyd passed away. In the ensuing years, whenever I heard the word "stroke," the conversation with him passed through my mind. When others experienced strokes I would share Floyd's words to reassure them that they weren't alone in facing the unexpected. They would often nod their head, as if to say, "No kidding."

Time passed.

Just over a decade later, as November 11, 2003, appeared on the calendar and a stroke came my way, it became my turn to live what Floyd could not fully say. In the ensuing days we searched for books that could shed light on the bewildering experience -- the way I "died" and could scarcely recognize myself; the way clocks no longer told the time; the way numbers no longer made sense and impulse lost the blessing of moderating restraint. We learned that strokes and Traumatic Brain Injuries (TBI) are cut of the same cloth. Strokes are caused by something that happens within the brain. TBIs are caused by something that happens to the brain from an outside source, a fall, an accident, or an IED in Iraq or Afghanistan. Both are now known as Acquired Brain Injuries (ABI). Both erase much of the way we once understood ourselves and made sense of the world. Both leave us wondering what the future holds. Neither simply goes away. We are left to navigate a new understanding of life.

It was not the first time I'd had such a challenge. As a Type 1 diabetic for nearly 50 years, I'd known about the ins and outs of diabetes since the age of seven. But as all people with chronic conditions soon realize, learning to accept an incurable disease is much easier said than done. When I shared with a doctor at Boston's famed Joslin Clinic that I had yet to come to terms with my disease after nearly 20 years, his diagnosis was unerring. "We call that acceptance," he said. "But how do you accept?" I asked. For that, he had no answer. It turns out that most of life's answers come not from the anticipated sources but from unexpected encounters. For me the key came from a woman who had been living with diabetes for half a century. "Live your life," she said. Her insight opened the door to acceptance and I soon began writing *Journey of a Diabetic* to share what I had learned along the way. I could not have imagined that living with brain damage made living with diabetes look easy.

A four word question, "How do you accept?" prompted my writing *Journey of a Diabetic*. Twenty years after its publication a four word question, "What's it like, Floyd?" again sought its story.

In the spring of 2004, after four months of rehabilitation, my wife, Connie, turned to Dr. David Gumm, a neuropsychologist at St. Vincent Healthcare in Billings, Montana and asked if he would be willing to write a book with us. She knew, with unerring wisdom and love, that finding something to do with the stroke experience was critical to both my recovery and my life. A doctorate in psychology and a post-doctoral fellowship in clinical neuropsychology, and a keen interest in what makes the brain tick, made David ideally suited to his work at St. Vincent Healthcare. Whenever he returned to the hospital after a professional conference, he could hardly wait to share what he had learned with both staff and patients. His enthusiasm and depth of concern for patients deeply blessed us all.

---

1 For a meaningful excursion into Descartes' thinking and its place in neurology, David referred me to, *Descartes' Error: Emotion, Reason and the Human Brain*, by Antonio Damasio, Putnam Press, 1994. Although it is not an easy read, it was helpful in understanding just what it is that neuropsychologists deal with when they work with brain injured patients.

"Yes," he said. He would be glad to lend his insight to our experience.

"Then let's start," I said. Several times a month David and I met over lunch and recorded our conversations. Neuropsychology was a new word for us. We knew about neurology and psychology, but had never heard of neuropsychology. To Descartes' dictum, "I think, therefore I am," neuropsychologists unfailingly and unflinchingly ask, "But why are you thinking that way?[1] Is it your personality? Or does it reflect the way your brain is scientifically wired? And how has brain injury changed that wiring?" Our personalities and psychological makeup depend on billions of neural pathways. When these networks are damaged, the way we perceive ourselves, each other, and even God, can't help but change as the crucial and beautiful relationship between perception and belief finds a new balance. Neuropsychologists gently, and patiently, tease the "tissue" of psychology from the "damaged tissue" of brain injury. It takes patience, compassion, and a consummate understanding of the way the brain works. While delving into the mystery of personality, neuropsychology invariably challenges conventional wisdom. In his book, *The Executive Brain*, Elkhonon Goldberg puts it succinctly:

"But if the neurological nature of impaired memory, perception, or language usually can be grasped by the general public, the executive deficit caused by frontal lobe injury almost never is grasped," he writes. "Point to the patient's impulsivity, volatility, indifference, lack of initiative, and the common response will be 'This is not his brain, this is his personality!' And the notion of 'personality,' of course, is something that, on a par with apple pie and spring water, carries moralistic, righteous connections. It is my hope [to] correct the unintended public insensitivity, and sometimes outright cruelty, toward the most devastating of all forms of brain damage, the damage to the frontal lobes."[2]

We eventually came to understand that the brain can be restored to new life thanks to the intervention and support of family, friends, therapists and even the hand of a seemingly absent God. With thanks to David and Connie, the words shared in the following pages are for Floyd and all who awake one day to find themselves in a world we can scarcely understand. May they shed light as we all find our way.

---

2 *The Executive Brain, Frontal Lobes and the Civilized Mind*, Elkhonon Goldberg, Oxford University Press, 2001

chapter one
a maple at fifth and mcleod

• • •

A maple stands at the corner of Fifth and McLeod in Big Timber, Montana. In late October, its leaves turn a magnificent yellow. Normally, they do not last long. Fall in Big Timber is a quick season, and the winds quickly blow away the leaves long before snow returns to the Crazy Mountains. Every once in a while, there will be a week or so when the wind fails to blow, when the fall colors have a moment to stand in stunning stillness under the clear blue sky, or beneath the brightly shining stars. When that happens, we can't help but notice.

So it was that walking to church one day the young maple caught my eye. Its branches were almost jet black, and its leaves were ablaze in Indian Yellow, whose brilliant light echoed between them. All of a sudden, several of the leaves let go. There was no particular reason, no wind, no passing car, no kids shaking the branches. They just let go and began fluttering to the ground. In a moment or two, hundreds of leaves joined the three or four that first fell. And then, almost before the newcomers touched the ground, virtually every leaf on the entire tree surrendered to the touch of fall. In a minute or two, the tree was bare and the ground was a pool of yellow leaves. During worship, when we gave thanks to God for the gift of life, I couldn't help but ask if anyone else had seen the leaves at the corner of Fifth and McLeod suddenly drop to the ground. "Yes," several said, they too had caught the unbelievably beautiful moment.

Brain injury is such a descent. All of a sudden, without warning, unexpectedly, neurons drop away. A blood clot suddenly blocks the sap that feeds the brain, that brings life-giving oxygen to its billions of cells. A fall, an accident or an explosion triggers the same thing. The brain begins to die.

For both the tree, and those whose neurons have fallen away, spring is many seasons away. The fallen leaves will never return; neither will the neurons. But in time, new leaves appear and the remnant neurons do what they can to pick up the cause of life. In neither case will it be life as it was. In both cases, new life must appear. There is, of course, a difference between a brain and a tree. Each fall trees are supposed to drop their leaves, sometimes with the help of wind, or sometimes of their own accord. Those of us with acquired brain injuries have rarely reached the season in our lives where such a loss is expected. For us, a stroke or brain injury is like a tree losing its leaves in mid-July. Suddenly, unexpectedly, the landscape of our lives changes.

There was a time in my life that I was somewhat fluent in French. Wondering what the word for stroke was in French, I came across *coup de cerveau* which means, "touch of the brain." Although *accident vasculaire cérébral*, is the proper medical translation, the more figurative *coup de cerveau* caught my imagination. Both stroke and coup are powerful words. At the stroke of a pen laws are signed, treaties are enacted, and wars cease. At the stroke of midnight something ominous occurs. We speak not just of midnight, but the stroke of midnight to name the exact moment of profound change. A stroke of insight comes as a sudden flash and the stroke of a moment condenses random time into a sudden point of transformation.

So it is with *coup*. A *coup d'etat* quickly changes a government, sometimes violently. Its touch will not leave the status quo alone. The coup de grace marks the end of a person's life. There is no recovery from a *coup de grace*. When Native Americans counted coup, it meant they touched an enemy and, in that quick touch, took power from them. Once coup had been counted, it lingered. The one who touched an enemy told the victorious story many times. The one who was touched rarely told the story that was, for him, a mark of shame. For both, the coup irrevocably changed the story of their lives.

When autumn counted coup on the maple at the corner of Fifth and McLeod, nobody could have predicted the exact moment its shimmering leaves would drop to the ground. Once they fell the iridescent pool of color around the base of the tree almost made up for the sadness of dark and empty branches. We were left to accept what happened as a natural part of life. We realized, as the poet William Stafford so beautifully wrote, "nothing you do can change time's unfolding."[3]

It was early in the week.

Church had been good that week. Exhaustingly and wonderfully good. As usual, I could hardly wait for Sunday. Whatever the Scripture might be, the stories and verses would inevitably be full of light and life. We would sing, pray, laugh, tease and shed an occasional tear. Each person had his or her own reason to sit in his or her chosen pew, giving thanks for life and asking for a word of divine guidance. The side room off the sanctuary would be used for overflow, while downstairs coffee, perhaps with elk sausage if one of the hunters had been successful, awaited us. We would sit around the tables catching up with each other, sharing stories until the cows came home. There were meetings, wonderful meetings where we'd think about Thanksgiving's approach, what we might do for advent that year, about mission trips to Paraguay or Jamaica, about baptisms and new members. "Church" was a word I'd come to love with every inch of my soul. Mondays were never days off, but always "catch up" days. The expression on someone's face on Sunday morning would signal the need for a visit, for a note, for a call. Sunday was the springboard for Monday's ministries. I was going full tilt, but that was nothing new.

I had no warning that the leaves of my life were about to fall.

I walked over to church as usual. Walking was a time to quiet the soul and breathe in the blessings of a new day. Early in the morning, when the mountains emerged from the shroud of night, and bathed them in soft crimson light, it always reminded me of the birth of our children when their blue skin ignited with that same light. On that Monday I made some calls, checked the messages, and tested my blood sugar as I normally did four or five times a day. A prick of the lancet produced a drop of blood that a meter read in a mere five seconds. For some reason my blood sugar was abnormally high. I took a corrective dose of insulin that should have brought me back to normal in a few hours. One can usually detect a high blood sugar without the meter. The body feels sluggish as the blood runs thick with sugar it shouldn't have. Fatigue presents itself. I took

3 **The Way It Is, New and Selected Poems**, William Stafford, Greywolf Press, 1998, p. 42.

some Humalog, a remarkably fast-acting and powerful insulin. Four units can drop a blood sugar 160 points in just a few hours.

Later that morning it was still abnormally high. I took yet another dose and waited for it to work. By two o'clock, I was inordinately exhausted and wanted to do nothing more than lie down. I walked home, stretched out, and took a short nap. When I awoke, I took yet another dose of insulin which also seemed to have no effect. Either I was ill, or something was stressing my body in ways I had never before experienced. It couldn't be illness. I rarely catch colds and the flu is something I've heard about but bypassed almost every year. "I don't get sick," I'd joke. "I go for the big stuff. I've made it through half a century of diabetes and two heart attacks. I don't mess around with colds."

Years ago, the logo of the Joslin Clinic portrayed a three-horse chariot with a single driver. The three horses were diet, insulin and exercise. Each one could influence the others. Controlling all three was essential to engage in the race of life. Any error, too much stress, too much insulin, too little insulin, too many calories, too much exercise, and we'd be in trouble in one of two ways:

Hypoglycemia is a very low blood sugar that induces the same symptoms as a stroke. A stroke deprives the brain of blood, hypoglycemia deprives the blood of its much-needed glucose. Although it makes up only three percent of the human body, the brain consumes between 20 and 25 percent of the body's glucose. A low blood sugar sows chaos into the metabolic system. A normally placid person becomes belligerent; balance gives way to stumbles and falls; vision blurs, sweating begins, and seizures wait to claim the day. Neurons are utterly unable to store glucose so supplying it to them throughout the day is a necessity. But I had just eaten breakfast, so that made hypoglycemia an unlikely culprit. If hypoglycemia wasn't the problem its equally pesky twin, hyperglycemia, could be the culprit. Hyperglycemia is a lack of insulin. Without insulin, glucose cannot turn into energy and the patient eventually dies. Perhaps I had not taken enough insulin — but five units of Humalog should have been able to handle anything. I had skipped lunch entirely, as I often do, so there was no way the high blood sugar came from too many calories running through my system. Stress, which tends to elevate blood sugars, seemed like a remote possibility. There had been no conflicted meetings, no upsetting phone calls, no sudden crisis to demand my attention. It didn't occur to me that my body was doing all it could to signal that something in my life was changing.

It was not the first time symptoms gave a warning without the blessing of words. On the eve of my seventh birthday I noticed I could never get enough to drink. Water ran through me almost as soon as I drank it. I quickly lost weight and food gave no strength. Something was wrong that took several weeks to diagnose. This time high blood sugars and fatigue sent warnings for a condition that didn't yet have a name.

It is one thing to describe a feeling--anger, love, resentment, hope--and quite another to find words for something that reaches into the very core of our being and has never been experienced before. Some might say, "Why didn't you ask for help?" We don't ask for help whether we are seven or 57 because we are so fervently holding on to life that the prospect of admitting something is wrong seems like a betrayal of life itself. And so we wait, we hold on, trusting that all will once again be well. It is not that we are in denial. When an unexpected veil begins to fall over our lives, we hold on and wait it out. And so I laid down and fell fast asleep.

Tuesday morning called for a seven o'clock meeting at one of the two coffee shops in Big Timber. For some reason I chose to drive instead of walk to the meeting. Prospector Pizza always gave our swimming pool committee a table around which we could talk about how to bring a swimming pool to a rodeo town. We had a daunting task ahead of us but figured if we cared enough and just kept at it, we'd someday have a swimming pool. I walked in the door and saw our group at one of the tables and sat down with them. We greeted each other with small talk and I tried to pick up the conversation's flow. It should have been easy. One person shares a thought, others respond, new thoughts arrive and are received with a smile or dismissed with a laugh. Meetings have their ebb and flow, and ministry is the art of paying attention to both. But that morning it seemed there were no opening places. For some reason the ideas were all disconnected and the voices all had a sharp edge. Three or four people were talking at once, but instead of blending together their voices collided with startling intensity. The waitress kept appearing with coffee or French toast or one distracting thing or another. Unable to catch the drift of the meeting, I became more and more agitated. "That will never work," I said to myself. "That won't either." A look of agitated distraction must have crossed my face.

"Larry, hello!" said Gail, from across the table. "Looks like you didn't get enough sleep last night!"

"No, I'm fine," I said. The senseless conversation continued, each word interrupting the thought beside it. I had no idea what we were talking about and wished I could hold the conversation at arm's length and stop the assault of sharp-edged thoughts and sounds.

Barbara, our public health nurse, remembers that morning well.

"You really weren't yourself," she later said. "When the waitress came to the table, she asked if you'd like a second cup of coffee. You said 'yes' and then she said, 'It might be a good idea if you took your thumb out of the cup.' It was both funny and weird. Something was going on, but we didn't know what." I always loved the folk song about the logger who stirred his coffee with his thumb, but nothing could have been farther from my mind than acting out the words of that song.

I lifted my thumb out of the cup, laughed a bit and was glad to sense the meeting drawing to a close. Perhaps it had been a sleepless night, but fatigue alone couldn't account for my incapacity to track the conversation or for the almost unbearably sharp sounds of the cafe. I had to get out of there. I paid my bill and went out to the unlocked car whose keys were in the ignition, where we always kept them. I opened the door, got in and took a deep breath. The car was mercifully quiet. I turned the key, listened to the engine turn over and slowly backed out. We park diagonally in Big Timber where most of the cars are trucks, often with a dog in the back end. Pulling out I felt the subtle presence of danger for the first time. Everything was happening too fast. I needed to slow down. Instead of driving onto the highway and navigating the traffic I turned into the bank's drive-up window lane which led to the shelter of an alley. The church was just three blocks away.

The road seemed remarkably bright. I covered one eye with my hand, and drove very slowly just to make sure an accident wouldn't happen. Once I made it to the church the sense of danger subsided. Time and insulin were both on my side. There was no need to call the doctor. Diabetics don't do that. We learn that we are in control of what happens to us, that we already know the answer to the doctor's predictable questions. High blood sugar—more insulin. Low blood sugar, less insulin, more food. It was the litany of life. The church office was quiet, its array of rarely read books was exactly where it should be, a watercolor painting of a mission trip to Jamaica was exactly where it had been for five years, the pieces of paper that mark the trails of ministry were exactly where I had left them the day before. I sat on the sofa, something I almost never did. The sofa was for families, for parishioners, for kids. It received me and my collapse. In a few moments I began to drift off to sleep. That was so unusual I decided it might be best if I went home.

We are a product of our genes; our experiences; our beliefs; our perceptions; our chosen professions; our families; and our various diseases. What word could possibly be more complicated than "self?" It is the brain that determines the answer to the riddle that asks if it is perception or belief that holds sway in our lives. It is the brain that finds the patterns; that makes or avoids the crucial choices; that fires billions of synapses to convey what we see; what we hear; what we think; what we know and how we respond to any given situation. We are who and what our brain says we are. Even our language underscores this.

"You're out of your mind," we'll say to someone who has suddenly taken leave of their senses.

Self. It is such an important concept that an entire area of the brain is devoted to identity. "It's lodged in the right hemisphere," David said as we talked about the November 11th of my life. "It makes sense that those were the difficulties you were having at the cafe. Had you had the same area of the brain in the left hemisphere, you probably would have been unable to talk, either slurring or not producing your words."

On the plastic model of the brain he uses to explain brain injuries to patients in Headway, the *rehabilitation* program at St. Vincent's Healthcare, different parts of the brain are labeled with their appropriate function. The words on the right side are so precious: Creativity; Initiative; Self-Awareness; Role; Abstract Thinking; Comprehension and Understanding. Taken together they spell identity and signify civilization.

Some of the zones on the right side are large, perhaps the size of a red plum. On the left side, the zones are smaller, resembling a line of multi-colored dominoes, each standing on end with painstakingly hand-painted labels on the edge. Each tag designates a function with scientific precision. Taste, sight, smell, speech, and hearing all have their place. A century ago a brain was just a "brain." Everyone knew it was essential for life but the idea that different parts of it handled different functions had not yet emerged. David explained that the breakthrough came as a result of the work of Wilder Penfield, a Canadian neurosurgeon who had been operating on patients with severe epilepsy. Brain surgery revealed itself to be utterly different from surgery on the rest of the body. No anesthesia is necessary when operating on the brain itself. The organ that reads pain in the rest of the body has no pain sensors of its own. As David talked it struck me how curious it is that it was also a Canadian physician who discovered insulin.

"After the skull was lifted away, Wilder's patients would be fully awake, and could talk with him," said David. "Wilder took a small probe and pushed it into different areas of the brain. When he placed the electrode in one place, the patient would say, 'Now I smell mother's apple pie.' When he moved it a bit, the patient might say, 'Now I taste a wonderful cup of coffee.' Another move might trigger a visual image or the memory of a sound. As he went along he noted the various responses in each part of the brain. Eventually, he had a map showing the parts of the brain responsible for its many functions. It was very, very fascinating work."

Although the validity of these areas cannot be denied, subsequent research revealed that these areas overlap, and that each area has a porous rather than a sharp boundary. Yes, there is an area responsible for smell, but the mysterious totality of a human being is complex, rather than simple. Memory can't help but accompany smell, sounds inevitably derive meaning from the voice of experience. As good as global positioning satellites are, their readings cannot describe a journey. Traveling from New York to San Francisco one passes through a million different positions. But a readout of those numbers will never tell the whole story—the sunsets, the conversations, the price of gas, the flat tire, the wind and the purpose of the journey. Essence is the work a hundred billion brain cells that perform at least one quadrillion operations a second. They do not operate in one simple way, but are remarkably fluid and mysterious in the unpredictable ways they convey information. A reductionist model simply cannot account for the essence of a human being, much less his or her soul. Neurology is not orthopedics in which the laws of physics and the capacity of a bone to mend are the two main players. Black and white thinking will not suffice for the complexity of a human being, for the essential perception of self. Logic alone is not enough, as Zeno pointed out two thousand years ago in his famous paradox that shows the limits of logic. When you reached for this book you cut the distance between your hand and the book in half. As your reach continued you cut it in half again. Whatever the distance it can always be cut in half. Even a billionth of an inch can be cut in half. By the rules of logic (but perhaps not the rules of calculus I have yet to understand) you would never touch the page you are touching now. Zeno reminds us that logic alone does not always yield understanding. Mapping the brain can be a good and helpful thing, but it cannot fully convey the mysterious entirety of life nor the unforeseen falling away of neurons on a November day. I slept most of the afternoon. When darkness fell across the sky at its early November hour I was grateful for an unconditional surrender to the healing rhythms of night.

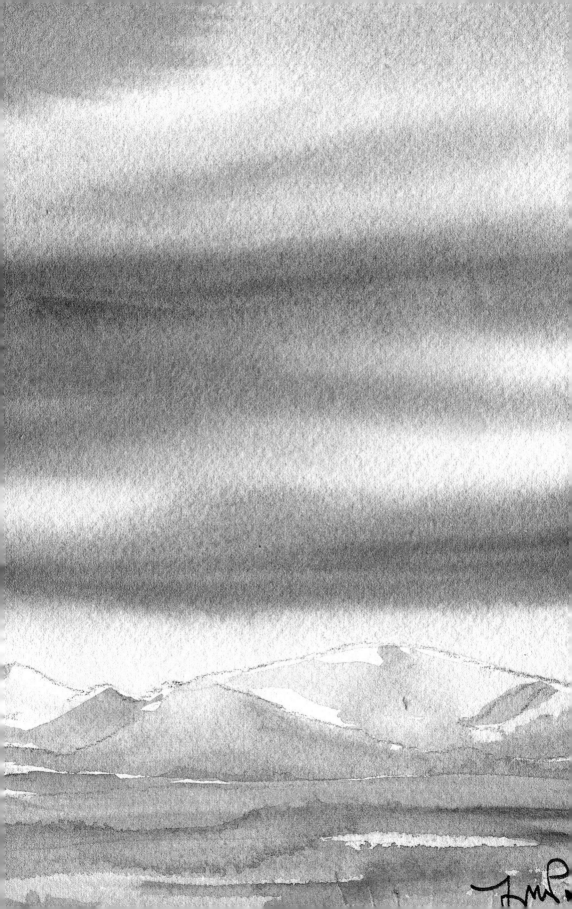

chapter two
dad?

...

Wednesday broke.

For most of my life, Wednesday mornings have been a time of fellowship. At seven o'clock, six or seven men gathered in the church kitchen for a Bible study while a corresponding women's book group met in my office. The arrangement was a true reflection of who actually holds power in the life of most churches. The women often shared their coffee with us as we met around the kitchen table and perused the texts that would form Sunday's sermon. I loved these midweek gatherings, the sharing of stories, the depth of fellowship, the easy conversation, and the appearance of both laughter and tears as we tried to make sense of life. To miss it would be unthinkable.

But when I awoke that Wednesday morning I knew I had to pass. "I can't go," I said to Connie. "I'm just shot, and I've got a headache." My blood sugar was sky high, as it had been the day before. She called the church and talked with Byron, who instantly knew something was amiss. He shared the message with the group. Whether they studied Scripture that morning or engaged in conversation, I don't know. I do know they drank coffee. I do know they saw the slip of paper that years before had been taped to the wall over the coffee pot reading: "Regular...½ cup; Norsk ¾ cup; Ultra Norsk 1 cup." I do know the Wednesday morning fellowship was as integral to their week as it was to mine. It was on Wednesday mornings that we shared our lives, our confusions, and the search for meaning and hope.

Connie was concerned. Headaches were not part of my repertoire. All those commercials about pounding headaches never made sense to me. To awake with a headache, and bow out of our morning get-together were sure signs of the gathering storm. She brought me some aspirin, and made a cup of chamomile tea. Sleep tried to claim the day but determination pushed it back. I got out of bed, made some coffee, and worked out on my garage-sale Nordic Track for 20 minutes as I did each day. I headed over to the church.

Mid-morning passed. I needed to be at the Legion hall to attend a funeral. In conjunction with hospice, I'd worked a bit with Larry and his family during the last month of his life. They opted to use the American Legion for the service. He had served in the armed forces, and many of his comrades in arms would be there. A pastor from his denomination would conduct the service and the Legion would present a flag to his family. Wanting to be there to offer support, I walked over and went up the well-known stairs into the auditorium. Sensing I was not up to carrying on a conversation with the many people I recognized in the room, I was glad to see a small island of empty seats at the front of the room. I chose one, sat down, looked over the funeral program and listened to the music. As I sat, the clot that dammed the flow of oxygenated blood to my brain continued to suffocate an ever-increasing number of cells, each of which took with it a shard or two of perception. My capacity to make sense of life faded as the neural leaves fell away. The parts of my brain served by other arteries kept running the same programs they had always run, but sensing something was wrong they also tried to pick up the slack causing my body to read "stress." No wonder my blood sugars were sky high. The clot was tiny, as most clots are, but it doesn't take much to block the flow of blood. Sixteen years earlier a tiny clot blocked the narrow channel of my left anterior descending artery, often referred to as the "Widow Maker." How strange it is that tiny clots can have such a far-reaching impact. And how strange it is that our vulnerability to clots is somewhat unpredictable. As a rule we rarely, if ever, ate fried foods. As a rule I exercised virtually every day, took two aspirin, followed a healthy diet and kept reasonable tabs on the decidedly unreasonable fluctuations of diabetes. And yet a clot broke loose from somewhere, traveled through a life-giving arterial system and finally lodged itself at a critical intersection. This time it bypassed my heart and found its way into my brain.

The speakers kept speaking, prayers kept rising, my sense of distance kept expanding. I couldn't connect.

"Why am I here?" I asked myself, startled at the bizarre question. "What's going on?"

"You know why you're here. You're a pastor," logic responded.

"Why am I here? How am I supposed to act? What is my role?" I wondered again. In my element, I was out of my element. The instincts that so unwaveringly told me who I was as a matter of faith, profession and call, had seemingly drifted away. It was almost as though I'd never been to a funeral in my life. When it was time to say the prayers, I said the prayers, but was utterly unconnected to the words. The Lord's Prayer sounded feeble and strange. I was operating on automatic pilot, something I'd promised to never do in a profession that demands authenticity as much, or perhaps more, than faith itself. When it was time to sing, my voice couldn't find the starting note. When it was time to greet the family, I wasn't sure what to say, what to do, how to connect. There were lines of people everywhere and countless conversations as people greeted one another and paid condolences to the family. I needed to break away.

Downstairs the Legion's Women's Auxiliary had prepared a luncheon for those at the funeral. I knew the room like the back of my hand. For over a century, our church served an election-day supper of creamed chicken, carrots, peas, pie and biscuits in that room. Over there is where we mixed and served the cranberry sauce. Over there is where the Hansen and Mack girls gathered up dishes, kept an eye on the pies. Nobody talked much about the election, whatever the results. This was time to break bread together, to enjoy a good meal and keep a tradition alive. I knew by name the people who prepared the ham salad sandwiches for the funeral luncheon.

"Larry, are you okay?" asked Edna, one of our church elders.

"Thanks," I said. "Guess I'm hungry." My voice was a dull and flat monotone. Normally, I would have asked them if they needed any help, or we would have engaged in the small talk that graces conversation between friends. But that didn't happen. As they went about their work, as people began to filter into the room, I felt utterly alone as my life continued its slow collapse.

"I knew something was wrong," Edna later shared with me. "You just weren't yourself. I asked if you were okay, and you said you were just tired, but I knew it was something more than that."

It was just a short walk from the Legion to the church. I opened the church door, looked again at the beautiful handmade fountain whose bubbling waters spoke of rebirth and looked up at the stained glass window we had custom made for the new church entrance we had dedicated at exactly midnight on the eve of the new millennium. Its dove with an olive branch portrayed a message of hope to all who walked in and out of the church. The sanctuary's stunning windows spoke silently and eloquently in the iconic language of light. There were many Sundays when I thought all we had to do was to gaze at the windows to find a heart-felt sermon. One showed a small boat about to set sail across the Sea of Galilee. We knew it represented the sea of life and that we too were called to cross to the other side in a small boat. We understood we could not get from here to there without storms that would threaten to engulf us. To the left and right of the large window were small panes of glass adorned with the symbols of communion: a sheaf of wheat and a cluster of grapes.

A few more steps and I was in my office. The chairs in my office were empty but full of stories. They were the chairs we moved to the front of the sanctuary for the confirmands after they shared their lives with the congregation in services that often brought us all to tears. The chairs faced a small, round table that centered countless committee meetings and counseling sessions. In its middle was a glass dish filled with red Paraguayan sand that surrounded a candle. Suddenly there was a knock at the door. As soon as I saw Tim and Melody's faces I remembered the appointment that had slipped my attention. They had asked me to officiate their wedding, which was only five months away. They didn't go to our church, but that didn't matter. We served a town, not just our members. I always loved working with couples as they prepared for their wedding. Premarital counseling always led to remarkably deep and honest conversations. I made it a rule to never even discuss the wedding details until we had talked about their lives, as individuals and as a couple, in considerable depth. I loved saying, "I'm going to give you a veto card. When arrangements start flowing too fast, and every aunt, uncle, relative and friend has an opinion about exactly how the wedding should be, and you begin wondering whatever happened to the simple notion of the two of you sharing your vows, I give you permission to say, 'That's a very nice idea but the pastor has to have the final say, and he tends to be very picky.'" They would always laugh, and so would I because we both knew playing that card might well be necessary.

I invited Tim and Melody in, trying to disguise the fact that I had completely lost track of the appointment. They sat side by side on the couch full of expectation and the unmistakable glow that surrounds newly engaged couples. The first meeting with a couple is an important one because it sets the tone for the ensuing sessions, to say nothing of the wedding itself. Although every couple is different, I had developed my own heart-felt script over the years whose words normally gave themselves easily, rhythmically, and meaningfully.

"Congratulations!" I said. " You've made a good and profound choice. There are no deeper words one person can say to another than, 'I love you, and I want to be with you for the rest of my life.' No other words come close to the life-changing power of a wedding vow. They will change you as individuals, and as a couple, not just now, but over the course of your lives. Our work over the next five months is designed to help you say them with complete clarity." They nodded.

And then I realized I had run out of words. The next phrase didn't give itself. There was an awkward silence. I wasn't connecting. What I had said fell strangely flat and I didn't know where to go. I reached for another phrase, sensing I was entirely out of step with the way these interviews had gone over the years. I wondered what to say next. A line I had used many times finally presented itself.

"There are three times in life that a person's name is said in a church in front of a group of other people. The first is when you are born, and the minister asks your parents, 'What is the name of this child?' The second is when you are married when the minister asks if you, Tim, will take Melody to be your wife, and if you, Melody, will take Tim to be your husband. The third is when we die and are commended by name into the hands of God. Each time is a sacred time. In marriage we even have a separate word that sets it apart from regular language. We don't call it a 'promise,' or a 'contract', or a 'commitment', necessary and worthy as those words are. Instead, we call it an exchange of 'vows.'"

Words left me again. I looked at them, explained we would need to meet five or six times for an hour and half or so each time. I explained I'd get to know them, and they would get to know me. Usually, this first session took at least an hour, but we had only been speaking 20 minutes or so. The unexpected lack of rapport made us all uncomfortable.

"You seemed really nervous," Tim later said to me. "And your face was kind of red. I wasn't sure exactly how church weddings are done, so I thought that maybe it was supposed to be that way." He was more than forgiving and as it turned out I was able to marry them six months later.

All day long I had been going on automatic pilot because something in my navigation system had gone wrong. Much later I learned about this curse of autopilot. When billions of brain cells are damaged or killed the remaining retain life's skeletal framework. Although it allows us to remember what 'should be,' we can't bring it to life or find a way to interpret it. Just as muscle memory tells a diver how to twist or flip, remaining memory cells continue to fire, trying to keep some semblance of order. Our brain injuries make it difficult, if not impossible, to perceive that there is no water in the pool.

One o'clock.

The second Wednesday of the month.

Our cancer group had a single mission. Its name was life. The medical system focused on diagnosis and possible cures, as it invariably does. But who would tend to life? Who would help patients learn to navigate the daunting intricacies of obtaining drugs that were far too expensive? Who would tease the demon of cancer back into its lair? Who would receive the tears of despair? Who would emphasize that living with cancer requires embracing life? Who would do so without issuing a bill? Who would do so without making church attendance a hidden obligation? Who would tend to healing?

We would. Our parish nurse fielded medical questions, answering why some drugs make one's hair fall out. A volunteer socialworker addressed the way cancer affects relationships. And I was present to share exactly what God had in mind when cancer decided to strike and stay. We were quite a group. Of all the centers of gravity that balance the life of a church, healing is perhaps the first as we seek to mend the world, our lives, and the diseases that come our way.

"What's up?" we'd ask. One person's story clarified itself as others shared their stories. Sometimes we used the box of tissues to wipe away tears born of sorrow, and sometimes we reached for them to wipe away tears born of laughter. Either way they were a mark of life. We met from one to two, knowing many would be too tired for an evening gathering, and tried to keep the sessions to just one hour though they frequently went a bit longer as one conversation gave way to another.

One day one of the members, Judy, brought in a hand-made quilt she had been working on as part of her walk with cancer. The quilt was entitled, Migration to the Light. When she unfurled it, we could scarcely believe its beauty. On a dark cloth were six colored squares. The red represented anger at the diagnosis of cancer. The green represented jealousy of those who had never had such a diagnosis. The black was despair. The blue square represented the all too few, but ever so meaningful moments of serenity. Towards the top the colors lightened, until one represented acceptance. On the background were thousands of stipplings that meandered seemingly without reason or purpose, but whose presence held the entire quilt together. Her quilt wasn't just about cancer, it mapped life itself and our inevitable migrations.

As the session drew to a close the phone rang.

"Hello?"

"Dad?"

"Hi Em," I said to Emily, our 22 year-old daughter. She was at Augsburg College in Minneapolis. It was not uncommon for her to call just to say hello. We had struggled over all kinds of issues, but it turns out that all the clichés about the bond between fathers and daughters are true. I remember her call but not the conversation she continues to carry in her heart.

"I remember walking from the enrollment center onto the quad," she later wrote. "It was fall, and everything smelled like leaves. I knew you were probably at church but had an urge to call you just to say 'hi.' You answered the phone and said 'hello,' and said you were with a group and couldn't talk just then. Normally I would have said, 'okay,' and called back. However, I know my Papa. Something in your voice was distracted, far away, not quite right. You were abrupt and distant. Even when you were busy you never sounded like that. I asked if you were all right and you just hung up the phone. That was weird. I called back. You hung up again.

"The third time I called back your voice was still more different. It sounded like you were talking in your sleep. To someone who knows you well it sounded silly, almost incoherent, but not playful. I knew something was wrong. I thought at first that you were having a bad reaction. Sometimes when you have reactions, they go so far you are in danger. I knew you wouldn't do anything about it in the middle of the group session. I called again and it was the same. You sounded sleepy and distracted. Your words were jumbled and not in the right order.

"I called the clinic and asked for Dr. Peden. The nurse said he was doing paperwork and would call me back. I told her I was a family friend and needed to speak with him right away. She put Kirby on the phone and I told him that something was happening to you. I told him that I thought it might be a reaction, but it sounded different than that, much different. I asked him to please stop what he was doing and check on you. He said he would and I hung up the phone. A while later Mom called me and said you were in the hospital."

I am still in awe of Emily's power of discernment and unflinching presence. It takes courage to interrupt a doctor and tell him what he must do. Intervention is a gutsy thing. And my daughter, our youngest child, my only daughter, had intervened.

The phone rang.

"Larry?"

"Yes?"

"Hey, this is Kirby. Emily just called and said things are off a bit."

"No, I'm fine," I said. He didn't buy it. The tone of my voice must have tipped him off.

"Well, why don't you come over."

"Now?"

"Yes, come on over now."

I may have said to him something about all the insulin I'd been taking, all to no avail.

"I'll be okay."

"Well, I think you'd better come over."

"Okay." The clinic was only four or five blocks away from the church. I went out to the car. Carefully, I drove south on Anderson, turned at the home of the family whose son I had just "counseled" regarding a May wedding, cautiously drove across McLeod, and on over to the clinic. I parked without a problem, and went into the waiting room. I've often thought that if I was a millionaire I'd give every waiting room a subscription to a dozen or so magazines just to keep the world up to date. When something is broken in your life there is something depressing about reading magazines that are three or four years out of date.

"Larry?" the nurse called.

"Yes."

"Come on back." I went into an exam room, and sat down on the chair.

"What's up?" Kirby asked.

"I don't know," I said. "Must be my diabetes."

He looked into my eyes, and noticed that my breath smelled fruity. That was a sure sign of too high a blood sugar. Ketoacidosis happens when the lack of insulin causes the body to burn fat instead of carbohydrates. It is frequently accompanied by a fruity breath. I was still certain that diabetes was the culprit. The disease that never goes away requires such constant vigilance that it is natural to make it the constant culprit. It can turn a small infection into a hospital stay, a good day into a veritable nightmare if the three-horse chariot of diet, exercise and insulin runs afoul.

I sat on a small stool while Kirby stood in front of me. A year later I noticed the poster on the wall full of misspelled words intended to show that mispronunciation is a warning sign of strokes.

"Have you been drinking?" Kirby asked. It was an absurd question, but an important one to discern with diabetes. People in reactions often look like, sound like and walk like drunks. My strange breath couldn't help but make him wonder.

"I just can't get my blood sugars down," I said. "Insulin is running through me like water." The words you see on this page deceive the way I actually spoke. "Blood sugars down" turned into "down sugar blood." I knew full well I wasn't saying the words correctly, and after they tripped me up I'd try to say it again, trying to get it right. My voice was a flat monotone.

More than that, my essence as a person was missing. Kirby and I had known each other for three years. I baptized him and their child, Luke, on the same day. Kirby was part of our church team that traveled to Paraguay where we participated in a work camp and set up a medical mission for children who rarely, if ever, saw a doctor. When I had been away on a sabbatical, Kirby and his wife Julie took over the confirmation program, working carefully and patiently with the young people. He knew me inside and out.

Rural medicine has its disadvantages. Specialists do not appear at the drop of a hat. There are no CAT scans, no MRIs, no steady supply of medications that might be rarely used. Our Big Timber hospital wasn't actually a hospital at all. Instead it was licensed as a Medical Assistance Facility that provides only low-intensity acute care and can keep patients for no more than three days. Patients requiring acute care must be immediately transferred to hospitals in Billings or Bozeman. Those who live in large cities with three or four healthcare systems view rural medicine as dangerous. Although statistics tend to be on their side, there are times when rural medicine has enormous advantages. One of them is a relational understanding of healing. Kirby took one look at me, and knew instantly that something was wrong.

"I know Larry Pray," he later said, "and the man sitting in front of me that day wasn't Larry Pray."

"I want you to answer some questions for me," he said. "What is the home country of the woman we worked with in Paraguay?"

I knew exactly who he meant. Renee Carter had been a missionary in Paraguay with her husband, John, for 35 years. Renee carried a Swiss passport, but spent most of her childhood in Uruguay. I've always had an impish nature when answering black-and-white questions, preferring to play with nuance. I wondered, "Should I answer Uruguay or Switzerland?" Both answers would be correct and either answer might get me out of the clinic.

"Sitzerland," I said.

But I hadn't said it right. I quickly corrected myself.

"No, SWITZerland," I said and then emphatically added, "
Not SITZerland. SWITZerland."

I spoke another sentence or two, once again mispronouncing the words, some of which came out in the wrong order.

"We need to get you to the hospital," he said.

"In Billings?"

"In Billings."

"I can drive it myself," I said.

"There is no way you're going to do that."

"I drove over here just fine," I said. "I'll be alright. Or Connie can take me," I no sooner said the words than I knew my argument was hopeless.

"No," he said. "We have to keep you monitored."

Then he looked down and said, "Larry, you could die."

At that point, my memory begins to fade. They must have led me to the emergency room and laid me on one of the beds. An IV line found its mark. An EKG was set up to see if perhaps my heart was involved. We lived just across the street from the Pioneer Medical Center. As soon as Kirby had stabilization procedures underway in the emergency room, and ruled out the possibility of another heart attack, he headed out the door, crossed the street, and walked into our house. Getting in wasn't a problem. Connie and I hadn't locked the door for years. He slid open the glass door and called out for Connie. Responding to the medications she must take to allay the pain that even her morphine pump can scarcely keep at bay, she was asleep upstairs. It was not unusual for her to take an afternoon nap to recover from the day's ever-escalating pain. When she didn't respond, Kirby opened the door, walked into the house, went upstairs found her asleep and gently reached over to wake her up.

"We've got to talk," he said. Connie had no idea what he meant at first, and thought perhaps something had happened to one of our children. They were all grown, but Kirby was still their doc, and if anything had happened to one of them he would soon know about it.

"Is it Emily?" she asked.

"No," he said, "but Emily called me. We don't know for sure yet, but I think Larry has had a stroke, or he has a brain tumor. He is in the emergency room, and we're going to send him to Billings just as soon as we can."

"Oh my," she said. He asked her a few questions, wondering how long I'd been ailing. She mentioned I'd stayed home from church and had a headache, which was unusual.

"I've got to get back across the street," he said. He had already called the neurologists at Deaconess Hospital, now known as the Billings Clinic, to let them know I'd soon be there. The much-touted clot-buster shot that can dissolve a clot and lessen the damage a stroke can cause is only effective if given within a few hours of the onset of the stroke. I suspect he knew there was nothing the shot could do. We had run out of time.

The ambulance crew arrived. I knew most of them and tried to talk, knowing what I was saying, even though the mispronunciations tripped me up. The ambulance was loud and smelled of exhaust as we pulled out of town. I wondered, in a teasing sort of way, how many people had asphyxiated on their way to the hospital because of those fumes. I kept asking where we were. Reed

Point? Park City? Laurel? The EMTs kept taking readings and asking how I was doing. That too seemed odd. It wasn't as though I was about to die of bleeding. I had no intention of dying.

We pulled into the Emergency Room at Deaconess Hospital. The EMTs and hospital crew lifted me from the ambulance, put me on a gurney, and wheeled me into a maze of fluorescent hallways. Connie and Karen, our church secretary, soon arrived. And then, not much later, Kirby and his wife, Julie, arrived. They, too, had driven the 80 miles from Big Timber to Billings, despite the hour. It was now nearly midnight. I was in one of those "rooms" that is defined by innocuously decorated drapes that hung by metal clips from steel tubes. It seemed the hospital was full and they didn't have a bed for me. We would have to stay in the makeshift room until a real room became available.

The neurologist Kirby had spoken with came into the "room." The expectation of relational healing that graces rural medicine quickly becomes a disadvantage when one needs to work with anonymous "big city" doctors who appear and disappear like puppets. They may save our lives, but they are not part of our life. Even when they try to be friendly, everyone knows that after the appointment is over the relationship ends. "Well, I hope I don't have to see you again!" they may joke. To have a doctor or a nurse you never see at the grocery store, the bank, in church, or at the gas station is strange. Trust and relationship are essential parts of healing but they are in short supply once you leave rural communities. I didn't know how to take this man in a white jacket who stood at the end of my bed.

"Do you know who I am?" he asked.

"No," I answered. How could I have known who he was?

"I'm the king," he said. He spread open his arms like an imperial ruler. My medical cubicle, the hallway, the emergency room, the entire hospital were evidently all his domain. In case I missed the point, he spread his arms in a grandiose gesture and added, "And all this is my castle!"

I didn't get it. I was glad to have Kirby and Julie there, and was so touched that they'd made the long drive. I was glad to have Connie there, and Karen, who would have to tide the church over during the few days I might be gone. The king left on an errand.

At some point, several of his subjects took me to another room for a CAT scan. I fit inside its tube just fine as they took a picture of my brain. After the CAT scan, they found a room for me on the telemetric ward full of patients recovering from heart surgery. The ward was familiar territory as I'd been there just five years before when I had my second heart attack. I was glad to be out of the emergency ward. The EKG meters were still hooked up; my insulin pump was still pumping, the IV continued to drip water into my veins, and people I knew and trusted were there with me.

The king returned. He came over by my bed.

"Your right brain is swollen," he said. He paused a moment before adding, "And that's not good."

Connie's diary preserves the day with succinct eloquence:

L woke up with severe headache again. Canceled 7 am prayer group! Gave him mint tea, took my meds, he got up after I went to sleep, the dog on bed with me, left phone off the hook on bed, Casey and me. Em called late am from Minnesota. L at church, said he sounded *very* strange. Actually hung up. Right hemisphere almost totally blank—blocked. New world. But Larry still with it. Thank God and all the spirits of the earth.

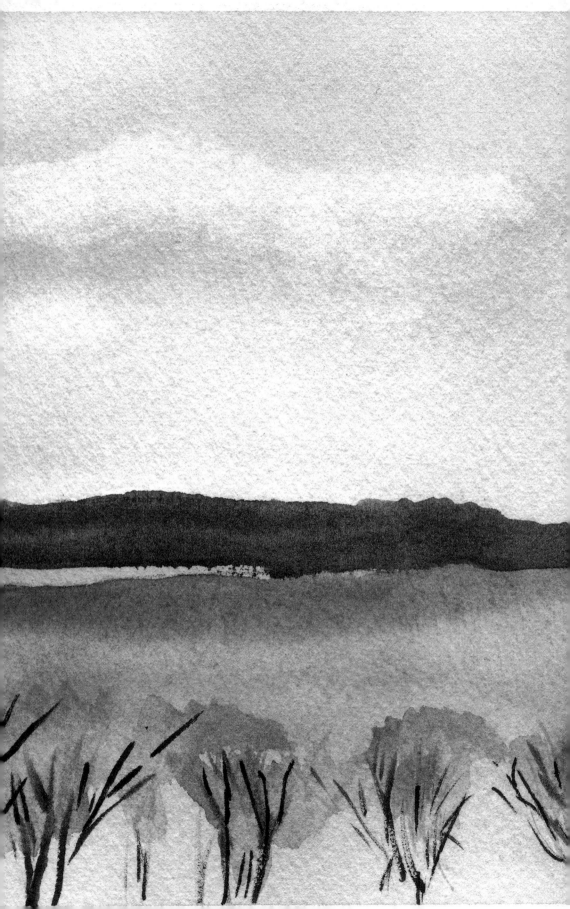

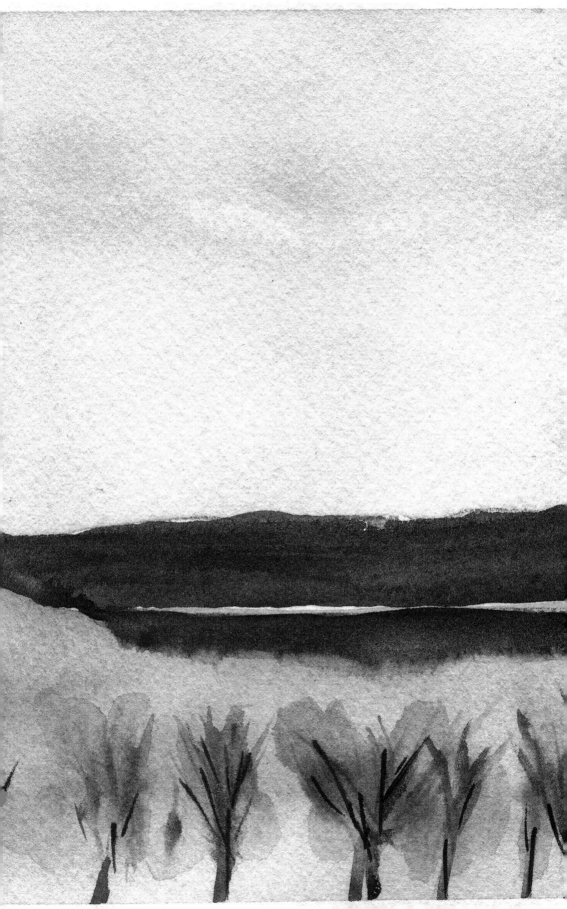

chapter three
tests

• • •

"Larry, you could die," Kirby had said. Now we knew why. The words were not frightening. We'd become accustomed to surviving. Neither of my two heart attacks had brought me down. Nor had diabetes per se, although its complications tried their best. For the moment I just wanted to get my voice back. I could still breathe, still stand, still see, but language and the relationships it blesses had fallen away as surely and silently as the maple leaves at the corner of Fifth and McLeod.

A broken-in jacket fits the body, gently shadowing every movement of its wearer. Soon it feels almost seamless. A well-worn glove fits when it follows the fingers' bends, or the top of a ski pole it grasps. It is all a matter of fit. And so it is with a human being. Our soul learns to fit our body; our body learns to fit with our soul; our personality frames the fit with gestures and expressions too numerous to count. We speak with our hands and glances as emotion crosses our face with expressions that can be universally understood. In music words fit the harmony, and rhythm fits both. When the fit is inexact we know it instantly. We awkwardly wear a new pair of jeans, and can hardly wait to get them home and wash them several times to help them find their fit. The salesman says, "Try this jacket." We try it on; put it aside; try another, put it aside, and in the end decide to not buy a new jacket, preferring the fit of the old one. As human beings, all is well when we fit. When we don't something is "off."

My words no longer fit. They belonged to somebody else.

My understanding of self no longer fit.

Emotions no longer fit.

I was alive but the blend of essence, soul, personality and history no longer fit.

"I'm okay, but it's not me" soon became the words I kept sharing with Connie, our children and parishioners who asked how I was doing. A different person inhabited my soul, my spirit, my body.

Words had been life's greatest blessing. They always had a way of giving themselves and finding meaning as though they had their own life. Sometimes they just appeared for no particular reason, and later root themselves in a poem or a sermon. Words touch all that makes us a human being. Each spoken or written sentence has the capacity to touch all that makes us human and all that makes us divine. It's not for nothing that one of the Gospels begins with the words, "In the beginning was the Word, and the Word was with God, and the Word was God." Nor is it insignificant that when God said, "Let there be light," there was light. It was language that powered creation itself. And it was my loss of language that took away the once coherent fit of spirit, self and soul and necessitated a new creation.

I could answer questions, but kept backwards getting the syllables. Words still gave themselves in thought but speech arrived as an awkward stranger. I was sure I could speak correctly if I just tried hard enough. But then, time after time "please" turned into "splease" and "Would you come back?" turned into "back you come would?" My voice was a drone. There are few words less human than "drone." The drone flies on without human touch. My voice was a drone; the person that wasn't me felt like a drone.

"I'm okay, but it's not me."

"Even without the CAT scan," said David as we unpacked my experience in the king's castle, "the loss of your voice indicated you had a right hemisphere stroke. We talk about the left side of the brain being responsible for language, and for the most part it is. But there is a component over in the right hemisphere that is responsible for the emotional tone of words, and even the emotional meaning of words. That's what you lost -- the ability to inject words with their emotional tone and meaning. You could say what you wanted to say, but you couldn't say it with the emotions you were feeling. When you think about it, that is what you did as pastor. Not only do pastors speak words, they must also convey the nuance and the meaning of those words in their tone of voice. And that's what you lost. When you say your voice was without lilt, that's exactly what the right hemisphere does. The nuance, the pitch, and the musical quality of the words had been taken away."

Connie was there, by my side, as she had been so many times during our 33-year marriage. She had been my support after my heart attacks, and each day as the stresses of diabetes took their toll. We had met at a mission agency in eastern Kentucky, working with children who had been abused or abandoned. The agency nurse warned her to not fall in love with me, as the complications of diabetes would be too much. To marry a diabetic was to ask for trouble. Connie didn't listen. We would find a way. At the time we had no idea she had a chronic disability that would be passed on to each of the children, and that I would look after her as much as she would tend to me. Either way, the purpose of life was to do something, and the purpose of marriage was to share it. I sensed as she stood by my bed that she was more concerned about my situation than I was. During the CAT scan she talked with the nurses, and tried to speak with the king, though it was difficult to get past the palace guard. Eventually she and Karen took a room in a nearby hotel, and Kirby and Julie headed back to Big Timber in the wee hours of the morning. I drifted off to sleep, unhindered by the fear that surrounded me.

"We're considering you a miracle," a nurse said the next morning.

"Why?"

"Well, you've had a massive stroke. It's hard to believe you can talk or move the left side of your body."

"Oh." At that point, the truthful diagnosis held no power. It had been different 17 years earlier when I went to an emergency room in New York City. For weeks I had been wondering why my left arm hurt, why my chest ached, why I couldn't find a comfortable position when I tried to go to sleep. Sensing from a thousand miles away that something was wrong, Connie asked a friend to convince me to go to the hospital. As I reluctantly checked into the emergency room and took a number, all I wanted to do as I waited my turn was to lie down on the green linoleum tiles and slip into a very deep sleep.

Finally a nurse called my number.

"Thirty two?" she said. I moved to the desk. "What's wrong?" she asked.

"I think it's my diabetes," I said. She asked me to lay down on a exam table. A few moments later a doctor arrived. He listened to my heart, reviewed my symptoms and asked the same question.

"Do you know what's wrong?" he asked.

"No," I said. "It must be my diabetes."

"No," he said with a gentle voice. "You're in the middle of a heart attack." At that point, a flurry of needles found their mark in the thin veins on my wrist and the deeper but hard to find veins of my arm. Had they asked me to lift my arm at that point, I doubt I would have been able to do it. It was a moment of complete surrender. Suddenly the chaos that surrounded me gave way to the coherence of diagnosis. Although I wasn't far from death, life made sense. I finally knew why I couldn't keep up with people as they briskly walked up and down the Broadway sidewalks. "How can they do that so easily?" I'd wondered. "Why can't I keep up?" When the doctor said "heart attack," the pieces of the puzzle fell into place. Suddenly we knew what we were up against and what to do. They wheeled me into the Cardiac Intensive Care unit, found the occluded artery, and scheduled an angioplasty.

It was a moment of surrender not only to the direction of the doctors and nurses and orderlies who suddenly surrounded me, but to God as well. It was not a heroic moment. Whatever would be would be, and that was okay. I did not have the strength to summon the will to live. I thought of Connie and our children, and the church that I had yet to serve, all in Minnesota awaiting my arrival. I'd been ordained just four days earlier, a ceremony complete with trumpets and organ, blessed by the presence of friends and colleagues. How uncanny it was to be ordained on a Sunday and then be in intensive care on a Thursday afternoon. In four days Palm Sunday's celebrations faded into Maundy Thursday's betrayal; in four days ordination anthems gave way to Thursday's broken heart.

"If I live, that's okay," I thought. "If I die. That too is okay. Either way, it will be well."

Years later, at a committal service on the outskirts of Dawson, Minnesota, a

Lutheran pastor read Scripture from Romans that echoed the sentiments of surrender.

"If we live, we live to Christ," wrote Paul. "If we die, we die to Christ. So whether we live or die, we are Christ's." (Romans 14:7-9).

"That's it," I thought. "That's what came over me in St. Luke's Hospital." Surrender can open doors that disease tries to close. It can calm the frantic winds of chaos and organize a coherent plan of action. But the word "stroke" held no such power. The word didn't latch on to any sense of meaning or lead to any hidden well of spiritual depth. The word felt empty -- interesting, but empty. It would take some time to comprehend what had happened during the days of descent as the leaves of my life fell away from their tree.

A nurse came in and asked me to draw a clock.

"Draw a clock?"

"Yes," she said, handing me a piece of paper and a pencil. It seemed like about the dumbest request I'd ever heard. I first drew a circle, and then put in the numbers. Heck, I could have done that in preschool, I thought. I didn't know that her request was a test that all stroke patients receive. If it's a right-brain stroke, some patients omit all the numerals on the left side of the clock. If it's a left-brain stroke the numbers on the right side of the clock may be missing. Curiously enough, they have no awareness that certain numbers are missing. Drawing a clock is a surefire way to diagnose what's known as "deficit awareness."

Another nurse appeared. She asked me to swallow.

"Swallow?"

"Yes." If drawing a clock seemed foolish, swallowing seemed even more so. She explained that some stroke victims have difficulty swallowing when that part of their brain has been damaged. So I swallowed. Anything else? I felt like asking.

Yet another nurse came into the room.

"Would you write something for me?" she asked.

"Sure," I said. At that moment, I decided to prove nothing had happened to my brain. I would write several sentences but they would not be in English. She handed me a piece of paper and I reached back to tenth grade English where we memorized the opening lines of English poetry.

Whan that Aprill, with his shoures soote

The droghte of March hath perced to the roote

And bathed every veyne in swich licour,

Of which vertu engendred is the flour…

I handed the paper back over to the nurse. She looked at it quizzically.

"Is this from Canterbury Tales?" she asked.

"Yes," I said. "Chaucer, Canterbury Tales." I'd aced the test. Nothing had happened to my brain that a bit of rest could not and would not heal. The clock had its numbers. The paper had its words. I had no inkling that my deficits would reveal themselves in other ways. I had absolutely no awareness I had survived the stroke that would allow me to live but had taken my life away.

"What caused the swelling?" I later asked David.

"Well, your stroke happened over an extended period of time," he said. "You first had one deficit, and then another, and then another, kind of like a slow avalanche. You had lost feeling in part of your body, that's why you could have your thumb in a coffee cup. Then you couldn't track conversations. Then you didn't know how to fit into the conversation. Then language began to slip. You had been hit by a truck, so to speak, and had been bleeding for days. When a clot blocked the blood supply to your brain and deprived the neurons of oxygen, they got sick, and that caused an inflammation. This happened in an area of your brain that is biologically extremely active. The neurons in the frontal lobe run in high gear all the time. They need lots of oxygen and lots of glucose. If they are deprived of either it doesn't take long for them to die. There are other parts of the brain that function in completely different ways. The cells in the brain stem that connects the brain with the spinal column never get geared up. They are like work horses that just plug along and take care of the basics like the heart beat or breathing. That's why some people lose the parts of the brain that allow for speech and perception and movement, and yet their hearts keep beating.

"Sometimes we'll see that when part of the brain swells, all of the brain gets squeezed and that results in a loss of oxygen. That's why a right-brain stroke doesn't affect just the right brain. The right brain swells but the left brain is also affected. And, of course, certain areas of the brain are much more vulnerable to that kind of an event because they are much more biologically active. The cells nearest the clot die first, and then as it progresses, you begin to get a massive deficit across the board.

"Fatigue is one symptom of this. And there's another factor at work. The brain is a huge energy user. When part of it is damaged, the other part has to work twice as hard to do what the whole brain did before. A lot of energy goes into repair. It leaves you feeling exhausted much of the time. What you could have once done without a hint of fatigue now leaves you utterly exhausted."

Different doctors kept entering the room. It seemed the "king" was away for the day, so one of his colleagues stopped by and asked me to hold out both arms. He held out his arms as well.

"Now pull against me using equal strength in each arm at the same time," he said. I did so as hard as I could. For most of my life, exercise has been a regular part of my life. For decades every morning began with exercise, usually a Nordic Track and some sets of garage-sale weights. I pulled as hard as I could. I would show him.

"Now draw up both your legs and push against me."

I acquiesced and did what he asked me to do not realizing how important those tests were. He wanted to ascertain the balance of strength in the two limbs. A right-brain stroke generally affects the left side of the body, leaving it weak or almost entirely dysfunctional. A left-brain stroke generally affects the right side of the body. They knew I'd had a right brain stroke, and wanted to test the strength on the left side of my body.

"That's amazing," said a nurse who had watched the push-offs. "You shouldn't be able to do that."

The first sign of the seriousness of my "massive" stroke became clear when our children began to arrive. Connie had called each of them and helped them make arrangements to come home. Tim, our eldest, found the first flight from Los Angeles where he worked as a Hollywood production manager. Emily quickly called together her friends and borrowed money to make the flight from Minneapolis. Ben flew in from Seward, Alaska, where he worked with the Big Brother/Big Sister program. His twin brother, Andy, was working as a television reporter in Cheyenne, Wyoming, and could not break free, but his call completed the circle. The three of them arrived almost at the same time. I could not believe they had made the trip. It had always embarrassed me as their father to never have the money to fly them home for a visit. Most kids flew to college; our kids took the Greyhound. As I used to joke with them, "Your friends will soon forget their flight, but you'll never forget crossing North Dakota on a Greyhound bus in the dead of a winter night." We would laugh, but down deep I'd be somewhat embarrassed. To see them, to hear their voices, to give them a hug, to sense the immediate presence, meant more than I could say.

From time to time yet another doctor would arrive. The doctor who gave the required prescription for my insulin pump stopped by, and Jan, the diabetes educator whose energy and care had come to mean so very much over the years, both provided the care that returned my blood sugars to a semblance of normal. In the course of a normal hospital stay there is a course of therapeutic action. If it's a heart attack, they find the clogged artery and then open it up or do a bypass. If it's a broken bone, they put in some staples or replace the hip, put on a cast, help you take the first few steps, and then tell you about how long it will be before life returns to its normal rhythms. If an infection is the problem, they take tests to find what the culprit is, and then add a small vial to the IV that drips into the saline solution until a cure begins to take effect. In other words, they do something.

But it appeared to me that nobody was actually doing anything. I didn't yet understand that neurology is basically a diagnostic science. Once they say, "It's a stroke," neurologists often leave the stage. I write these next sentences carefully and somewhat regretfully, aware that the patient's perception of medical care is often deeply askew. Much of the care physicians try to give is crowded out by the patient's stress, misunderstanding, and sometimes the condition itself. If a brain-injured patient cannot understand, it is a sure thing he or she will not understand. By the same token, much of what we have to share often fails to register in the course of a ten or fifteen minute exam. In the midst of it all, a chasm appears that blesses neither patient nor practitioner. In modern medicine the science of diagnosis often eclipses the art of forming healing relationships.

Neurology is especially vulnerable. Its practitioners specialize in finding and pinpointing what's wrong. They are the ones who say, "Your brain is swollen." There is money to be made in such diagnoses, but little money to be made during the years of life's quiet return. Although neurosurgeons can take out a tumor, or operate on one part of the brain or another, neurologists as a whole excel in diagnosis rather than healing. We eventually leave the hospital on a blood thinner that might preclude another clot but we do not leave headed toward a cure. I was anxious to have Kirby be my doc once again.

Finally, one nurse or another shared with Connie and the kids that there would be two tests performed by a department that already had reams of files concerning my life. My second heart attack had happened just three years before the stroke. In the middle of the night, with an aching arm that once again signaled an impending crisis, I had walked across the street to the emergency room and said I knew what those symptoms meant. They loaded me on a helicopter that flew me to Billings. I'll never forget arriving at the heliport and looking up into the black November sky as they wheeled me in from the hospital roof. I'd never seen a night sky with such deep absence of light. In Hebrew the word for "darkness" in the first lines of Genesis actually means "deep darkness." For the first time, I gazed into the full meaning of that word. They soon found the occluded artery, and immediately placed a stent in the "Widow Maker."

This time the cardiologists wanted to determine the source of the clots that had wreaked such havoc in my brain. Frequently, clots form in the carotid arteries that run up the side of the neck and on into the brain. As one ages, these arteries are prone to clog up. In fact, it is not uncommon to have them reamed out to make sure a stroke doesn't occur. The cardiology team arrived, gave me a sedative, placed tubes down my esophagus, and took a picture of my heart and various arteries. Mercifully, just as they said would happen, I woke up with no memory of the procedure itself. The good news was that they didn't find anything unusual. They saw the damage from my first two heart attacks, but didn't seem concerned. Four months later, with 20/20 hindsight, Connie and I wished they would have been far more concerned.

The other test was an MRI. I knew this one would be duck soup. All you do is lie down, get pushed into a tube, hear a loud clanking noise, and wait for the results. The gurney arrived. The MRI center wasn't in the hospital itself. It was in a separate building just a stone's throw away. I could have easily walked and wanted to show them I could. But they said no or, more likely, probably their insurer would not allow it. They wheeled me out of the hospital and put me in an ambulance for the 50-yard drive. I kept wondering how much that ambulance trip would cost. If they would have let me, I would have walked. But that was a "You've got to be kidding" kind of thought. We arrived virtually across the street, and they pulled me out of the ambulance, placed me on yet another gurney, pushed me into the waiting room and said it would be a short wait.

"That's fine," I said. The waiting room was actually a small office with several shelves of medical texts. One thick blue book caught my eye immediately. It had the look of authority. I pulled it from the shelf, and leafed through it. Its pages described virtually every condition known to humankind. I decided it would be a good time to learn something about this word "stroke." Sure enough, there were some pages devoted to strokes, complete with diagrams, pictures and paragraphs written with incomprehensible words. In one way or another, the reference book knew what I needed to know, and so there I sat in my hospital gown trying to learn what had happened to me and what I might do to turn the tide.

It is amazing that as we age we realize we actually don't change much at all. When I was seven, I decided after a few days of having nurses and my mother give me the first life-giving shots of insulin that I needed to be in charge. "I can do this myself, Mom," I gamely said. And so I did. This time I didn't reach for a syringe but for the medical books with the ever-ready determination that I could overcome whatever the obstacles might be.

A nurse eventually came into the room and said it was time for the MRI.

"Okay, let's go," I said returning the heavy book to its shelf, and following her into the room. Everything went just as predicted. They told me to stay very still, and assured me that they'd be able to talk with me on a little sound system, and that the test wouldn't take long. They'd get pictures from all angles and an injected dye would provide contrast to create a sharper image. Everything proceeded without incident. When it was over, they wheeled me back to the loading area, and an ambulance arrived. I wondered if I'd be billed for two ambulance trips that day. Back at the hospital, Connie, Tim, Ben and Emily were waiting. Their presence was a blessing, and my pride in our family was immense.

At one point the king stepped into my room. I asked him if I could return to work.

"Sure," he said. "You can go back to work full time after a week or so of rest."

"Great! And what about my morning workouts? Can I exercise again?"

"Yes," he said. "No problem."

Connie was flabbergasted.

"Do you know how hard he works out?" she asked.

"It's okay," said the king.

"Well, that's good news," I said. "So when can I go?"

"It won't be long," he said. He left, and I never saw him again. The next day his colleague stopped by and emphasized that I should neither go back to work nor return to a full-tilt exercise program before two or three months had safely passed. What he said didn't register. I had heard what I wanted to hear. My brain knew how things had been and therefore knew how things should be, and would not be hindered by unwelcome truths.

It doesn't take long to read a MRI. Radiologists are on call, and usually, within four or five hours the neurologist or doctor can view it either on a huge sheet of negatives or on a computer screen. The nurses kept saying I was some kind of miracle, and that the stroke had indeed been massive. Later I learned the word "massive" is a bit misleading. For some people, an MRI shows that just one small area of the brain has been affected, but loosing that one small area is enough to disable an entire life. Others might show a larger impacted area but for one mysterious reason or another, these patients function just fine after a few weeks of rest. "Massive," in terms of area does not always mean "massive" in terms of damage.

As I slept one afternoon, Connie and the kids tried to arrange a meeting with a neurologist. They wanted to know what the MRI had shown. The consultation, however, seemed virtually impossible to get. The stroke coordinator couldn't arrange it. The neurologist on call didn't have predictable hours. There is a tipping point in modern medicine when the patient's family becomes acutely aware that their pursuit of information is an unwanted distraction to those who can provide that information. The higher and more expensive the specialization, the quicker the tipping point seems to appear. We were eager to return to our no-stoplight town whose docs found the time to field the concerns of a daughter, and would walk across the street to say, "We've got to talk." Without their heartfelt presence we would have been truly alone in the high-tech medical wilderness.

It had become apparent that nothing was happening in the hospital that could not happen at home. Besides, there is nothing as depressing as vegetating in a hospital bed. My heart monitors were still hooked up. The screen indicated that every so often an untoward blip appeared on the screen, but there was nothing to do about it. They had told me that if I left the floor one alarm or another would sound. Stroke patients are a bit like Alzheimer's patients in a nursing home who take to wandering. For years I'd said that if I am ever admitted to a nursing home I would be a wanderer, an escape artist, a traveler. One of my dementia-ridden aunts once said to me in her nursing home, "I have a secret plan to get out of here. I just don't know if it will work." I smiled, hoping I'd have the same thoughts if I was in her situation. "It's a big world out there," Connie had once said to me. She was right and nothing could be worse than confinement. No matter what they said, I wanted to go home. I got out of bed, walked through the ward door and headed down to the hospital cafeteria. All of a sudden alarms went off and two nurses came running after me.

"Where are you going?"

"Down there," I answered pointing to the cafeteria at the bottom of the stairs.

"No, no, no, you must go back."

"Dad, what are you doing?" asked Ben.

"Leaving," I said.

"Dad, you can't do that."

"Okay, okay."

I went back to the room, tired, anxious, chastised and eager to put the day behind me. Although Ben and Connie understood that the impulsive behavior and lack of judgment were a result of the stroke, I had no such understanding. Right-brain strokes take time to reveal their full implications to the patient. It takes time for the mispronounced word, the misspoken sentence, the drone voice and the loss of rapport to reveal that they are but the tip of an iceberg. Right-brain stroke or TBI survivors seem just fine at first, but talk with us for a while and deficits begin to appear.

It never occurred to me that one of them would be the substance of faith itself.

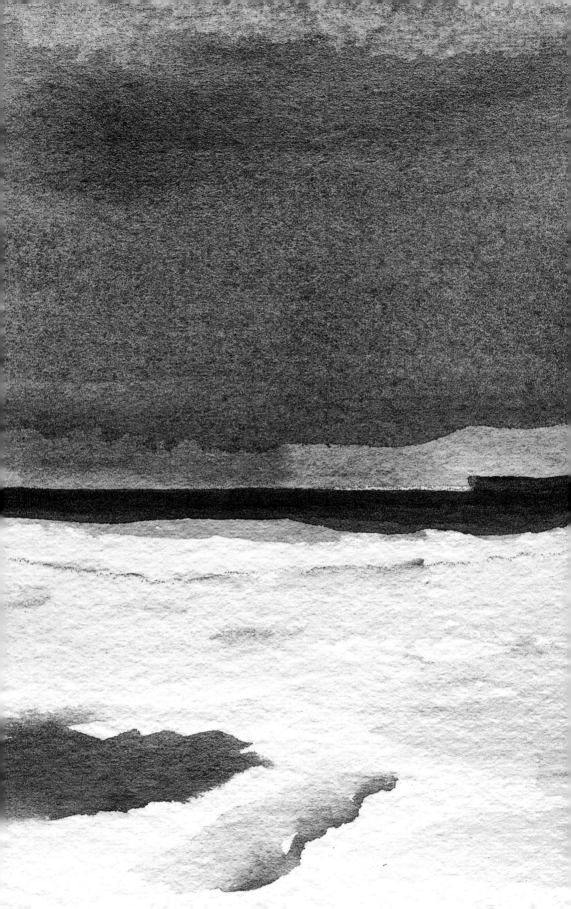

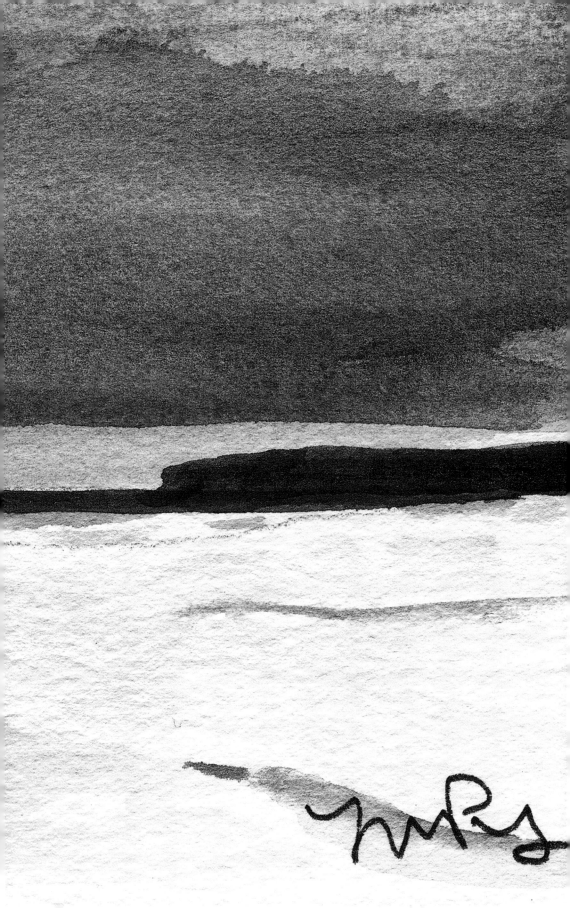

chapter four
disappearences

• • •

Connie had called our minister, the Rev. John Schaeffer. The United Church of Christ does not have bishops, but we do have Conference ministers whose calling it is to care for clergy and the churches they serve. John served as pastor to our 32 churches thinly stretched across Montana and Northern Wyoming. He had stood by us through thick and thin and we had stood by him. She didn't have to ask him to pay a visit knowing he would be on his way just as soon as he could arrange it. I greeted him as he walked in, told him that I'd somehow defied the odds, and that soon I'd be going home. John took in what I'd said, weighing it against what he had heard from Connie's report. John was not an overly effusive man but he always took ministry to heart. The fact that he kept confidences and considered carefully all that he heard was part of his strength. Ideology was not part of his theology.

After we'd spoken a bit, he leaned forward and asked if he could say a prayer.

"Sure," I said without thinking. I had said a prayer with Floyd after his stroke, now John would share a prayer with me after my stroke. Prayer is what pastors do.

One summer I was high on a scaffold painting the church eaves. The scaffold was safe, but we needed to use its third tier to reach the peeling paint beneath the eaves. I am not especially afraid of heights but the thought of losing balance up there was anything but hidden from consciousness. There was nothing to hold onto, no branch, no rope, no ledge that might save me from a fall. I noticed that all I needed to do to reassure a sense of balance was to gently touch the eave with my free hand. The light touch could not have saved me had the scaffold suddenly collapsed, but it provided a reference point sure enough and reassuring enough to save a fall. Prayer is like that, I'd said to the congregation. It is the reference point that keeps us from falls. When we pray privately, or when we pray as a congregation, fear subsides and we regain balance.

Then, to my utter astonishment I added, with a slightly caustic tone, "You'll have to do it yourself." My words had a sharp edge.

Prayer had been a friend. Sometimes it was in front of the church. Sometimes it was in silence. I had always loved the insight of St. Francis who once said, "Pray always. If you have to, use words." But although prayer had been part of my life, something had changed. At that moment the thought of prayer seemed impossible. Prayer had nowhere to go. Neither did God. God had vanished.

In the world of pseudo-psychology, it would be tempting to say, "You were angry at God, weren't you?"

But such an observation would miss the mark. The notion of being angry with God for almost anything had never been part of my life. There is nothing even faintly heroic about that sentence. It just never occurred to me that being angry with God for something that happened in life made much sense. Diabetes had taken insulin away, but it didn't take life away. During my heart attacks it wasn't anger towards God that propelled me, it was an acceptance of God's enduring presence that set the stage for healing. Yes, God is much better in the restoration business than he or she is in the prevention business, but such an observation didn't lead to disillusionment. Anger at God's being slow to arrive had never characterized my life.

I had always thought of God as the creator who birthed order out of the chaos. I once had a kaleidoscopic poster with the many names for God. Among them were Bright Morning Star, Author and Finisher of Our Faith, Prince of Peace, and others. For me God's name could have been Help, Comfort, Mercy, Justice or Grace. One of the Hebrew names for God sums it up best: *Chaim*, which means "Life."

The hymn, *When Peace Like a River*,[4] reflected both my theology and the seminal experiences of my life:

> When peace like a river, upholds me each day,
>
> when sorrow like sea billows roll,
>
> whatever my lot, you have taught me to say,
>
> it is well, it is well with my soul.

4 When Peace Like a River, by Horatio Spafford, *The New Century Hymnal*, Pilgrim Press, Cleveland, Ohio, 1995.

When John asked if we could pray, all of this had washed away. In seminary, I had taken a class taught by Roger Shinn, a remarkably sharp and caring Christian ethicist whose books unpacked the layers of meaning found in the Sermon on the Mount, and the streams of ecumenical thought that constituted the United Church of Christ. The class was entitled "Perception and Belief." Do we believe what we believe because we perceive it? Or do we perceive what we perceive because of our beliefs? Which is it? How do these two worlds work together, and what happens when they clash? Did the grounding capacity of prayer emerge from the world of perception? Or was it spawned by belief? And what happens when the brain responsible for both is struck by a stroke or TBI?

In *Hamlet*, King Claudius tries to pray after killing Hamlet's father and marrying his mother. His actions had caught up with his conscience, and made it impossible for him to pray. As he put it, My words fly up, my thoughts remain below. Words without thoughts never to heaven go.[5]

For prayer to be meaningful there must be an intimate connection between words and thoughts. As John took my hand, that connection was nowhere to be found. I thanked him for coming and lay there, thinking how strange my response had been. I tried in the silence of my thoughts to send forth a prayer to the God who had lovingly sustained so much of my life. It was no use. Both thought and words lacked a compass.

God had vanished. During my heart attacks I could surrender and trust that all would be well. But this time there was nothing to surrender to. If I had once perceived deep darkness as the source of creation itself, now there was no color at all. Even the age-old notion of being "lost" and then "found," made no sense because it depended on some sort of relationship, on some way to measure spiritual distance.

"May we pray?" John had asked.

"Okay, but you'll have to do it yourself," I had responded.

The holy had washed away.

---

5 William Shakespeare, *Hamlet*, Act III, Scene III

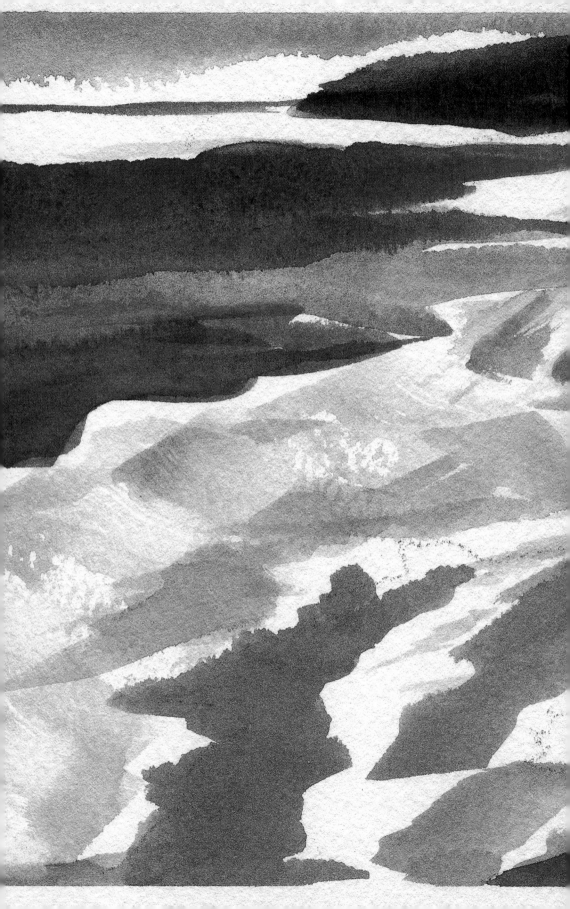

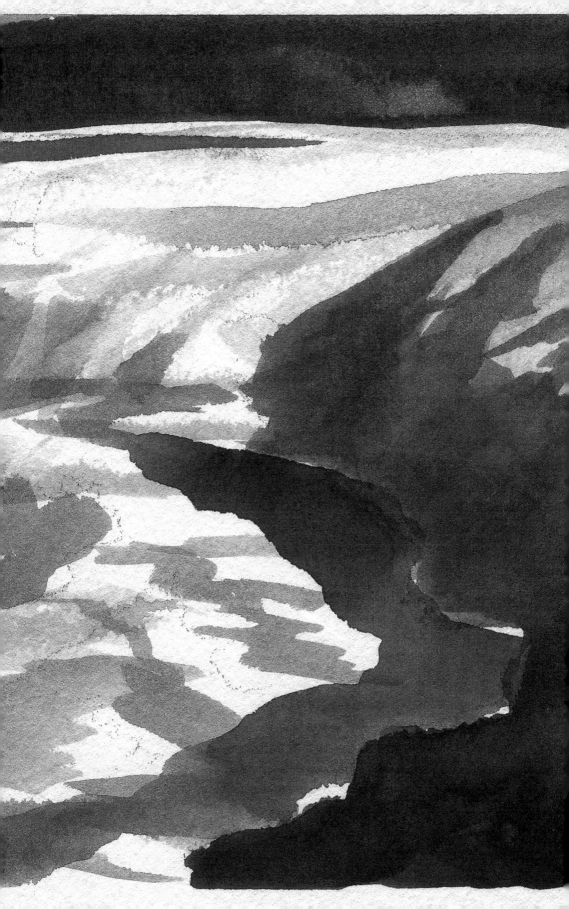

chapter five
flooded

• • •

It's odd how rarely we think about the brain. We are far more aware of the traffic it carries than the city it constitutes. We've heard that all roads lead to Rome, and we may have learned in high school biology that all nerves lead to the brain. We know the optical nerve transmits the gift of sight, but easily forget that countless other neurons tell us what it is we have seen. We know it takes thought to pay attention to a conversation. We know we need a rest after too much cramming. We're not quite so aware that it is the brain that transforms the striking of a piano key from sound into music, and then, perhaps, music into a sacred dimension known as art. The "feel" of music is a product not of the hands but of the brain that allows for phrasing, for lift, for rhythm, for a subtle differentiation of sound that transforms a sequence of symbols on a musical clef into sublime music. Our common knowledge of the brain is sometimes limited to Roadrunner cartoons that show what happens when a head is hit too hard. We laugh at the ensuing confusion and smile when the resulting stars appear. But for the most part we don't give this knowledge much power.

The French philosopher René Descartes transposed a seemingly mundane observation into a theological premise when he noted that thought constituted the very core of one's being. As he said, "I think, therefore I am." Take away the capacity to think, the capacity to order the world, and you have stripped a person of his or her essence. Strip away the billions of brain cells responsible for abstract thinking, for comprehending the Holy, for discerning beauty in both the mundane and the sacred in big and small events, and soon life and spiritual essence slip away.

"May we say a prayer?" a pastor had asked a pastor.

"Okay, but you'll have to do it," came the disconnected and inappropriate reply. In time, I began to realize how incredibly vulnerable we are. Parts of our lives that once seemed rock solid were no more than a mysterious network of several billion cells. I do not mean to imply that our perceptions of God are a trick that is manipulated by a chance arrangement of neurons. But I do mean to say that our perceptions of truth are guided by experience, and we can only draw from experience when our brain makes sense of the millions of messages it receives in the course of everyday life. The brain makes sense of the three relationships that constitute life: God, self, and neighbor. Confucius pointed out that establishing and maintaining right relations holds the key to life. He could not have known that doing so depended upon the neural networks of the right brain. It is responsible for both connection and coherence, perception and belief.

The day of departure arrived. A few more hospital meals. A few more instructions from one nurse or another. Words from yet another neurologist urged me to disregard the instructions of the "King" and emphasized that I would not be back at work in just a few weeks.

"Take it easy," he said. "You'll need at least a month."

We signed a few forms, packed up my belongings, left the hospital and headed for home. Once in the car, we decided to stop at a store to pick up a few groceries. When you're in the big city, despite the tinge of guilt about not shopping locally, picking up a few things is what small-town people do.

I sat in the front seat. Connie pulled onto Grand Avenue, one of those could-be-anywhere roads filled with traffic, lined with bright signs each claiming attention and each unlinked to anything but its own enterprise. We passed a little strip mall. A gas station. An oil change business. A car dealership and a piano store, a health store, a bike shop. An Army-Navy store and an Electronic Tax store. It all rushed by at breathtaking speed. I could scarcely keep up with the rush of events. What had always been a simple single task - drive down the road; find a store; turn in; go in and pick up some groceries - turned into a maze of the light, sounds, sights, movement, and the traffic. Finally the supermarket came into view. We pulled into the parking lot. Connie and Karen said they would be in the store for just a minute or two, but I had no intention of staying in the car. One doesn't celebrate being out of a hospital by staying in the car. And so, the three of us walked into the store.

Like most grocery stores it had an automatic door. You don't do a thing and it opens, ushering you into the cornucopia known as a "supermarket." Connie and Karen moved to the parts of the store they wanted to see, and I decided to mosey a bit down another aisle. I stepped past the cash registers and felt slightly sick. The scanners kept beeping. I'd never heard them so loud and chaotic. A display of brightly colored cartons of soda seemed on the verge of collapse. Every item on the shelves begged for recognition. Everywhere people were moving. Everything called for decisions. The lights were bright. The sounds were sharp. The people many.

Pastors frequently turn to scripture when they describe their lives. I've always loved the word "flooded" to describe an overwhelming situation. One can be flooded by a wave of emotions just as surely as 40 days and nights of rain. Standing in that store there was no doubt about it -- I was flooded, and the ark still had 80 miles to travel. There were too many things happening at once. Most enervating of all was the realization that everybody else in the store seemed to be doing just fine. They went about their motions effortlessly. I was the only one who couldn't keep up. Finally, Connie appeared and I told her I needed to go back to the car.

"It's too much," I said with a sense of panic. Real life had an abrasive edge the hospital's confines had successfully kept at bay.

We went outside and found the car, thankful for its safety. A blanket of fatigue spread through my entire body. We couldn't get home fast enough. Maybe the stroke had taken a toll after all, a toll that transformed a grocery store into a gauntlet.

"Damage to the frontal lobes of your brain accounts for this," said David as we reviewed the day. "You know, in any social situation, there are thousands of things a person could do. Most of them are immediately filtered out. You have to do that to come up with the best choice. For example, you could have bought every single item on the shelves of the grocery store that day, but you didn't because the frontal lobes instantaneously ruled out that possibility. What it couldn't filter out that day were all the sounds, all the sights, each of which begged for a response of one kind or another. That's what you found overwhelming.

"Think of the frontal lobes as the conductor of an orchestra. If the conductor dies or doesn't show up for a concert, you still have the violins and the brass and the percussion section, but they don't know when to come in, or how to play together to make a coherent sound.

"Or think of it this way. You have a probability generator up in your frontal lobe. In any situation it is always calculating the best response, and then it goes one way or another. Each possibility is on a kind of video cassette. You plug in that cassette, and that behavior comes out. What your brain does is to select the best cassette to play at any given moment. But what happens next is curious. Instead of stimulating that one option, your brain works to inhibit all of the other options and that leaves only one possibility. The vast majority of neurons in the frontal lobe are inhibitory in nature. They are governed by gamma aminouyteric acids. These neurotransmitters inhibit everything except what needs to come out. Making choices is actually an elimination tournament.

"When you were in the store, because your frontal lobes were damaged, you could not filter out what should and shouldn't happen. Everyone else in the store could do what they were there to do, and they were oblivious to the thousand possibilities that might have pulled them in other directions. But for you, every light, every color, every sound, every interaction presented itself as the one and only thing happening and yet they were all happening at once. No wonder it was overwhelming. The filter that brings order to countless thoughts and perceptions had been badly damaged in your stroke. That's why you needed to get out of the store, into a place where there wouldn't be such a rush of perceptions. And that's why you wanted to go to sleep. You needed rest at that point, and your body needed desperately to limit what your brain was taking in. No one can live in a spinning world. And that spinning was maybe the first physical sign that yes, you had in fact had a massive stroke and, yes, you had in fact been hurt far more than you thought."

We talked for a bit in the car. I must have looked ashen because I could feel both Connie's and Karen's concern to get home quickly. Karen had been a hospital administrator and had seen the toll strokes had taken on many people over the years and I could tell she must have talked with Connie about the life-changing implications of a stroke. I nodded off to sleep, waking up when we finally drove into town. The mountains were as beautiful as always. Our dog, Casey, a Springer Spaniel, who slept on my shoes whenever I was away from home, jumped and barked as we walked through the gate. The door sounded exactly the way it had a thousand times before when we pushed it open. The house with its paintings and rugs, its pictures of the kids, and its beautiful bouquets of flowers that had been delivered by various members of the church seemed so safe, so familiar. Everything was in its place.

I went upstairs, laid down, and fell asleep almost instantly. Usually sleep is a blend of physical and mental exhaustion. But this first at-home sleep had a different quality. It was a matter of complete surrender. My body craved rest. Before the stroke I might have said, "Gee, I'm tired tonight. It's been a full day." Now there was scarcely strength for such a thought. Instead, it was a complete collapse into the serene depths of oblivion. Sleep held chaos at bay.

Almost 12 hours later I awoke. For years my mornings had always been the same. I awoke, went downstairs, turned on the radio to hear National Public Radio's Morning Edition, and went over to my Nordic Track and began a workout. Twenty minutes of the Nordic Track led to another 20 or so minutes using one or another weight machine we had picked up at one garage sale or another. I've never been a fitness fanatic, but had always believed that exercise was the best way to avoid the daunting complications of diabetes. If I was to see, if I was to avoid heart damage, or if I was to survive heart attacks, I had to exercise. The fact that my antidote hadn't worked didn't dissuade me from staying in a semblance of shape. Regular morning workouts set the stage for the day.

And so I did my workout, and then had a light breakfast. I wanted to go over to church and pick up where I had left off. Connie's wisdom prevailed, however, and I began to just quietly spend the morning reading the mail, wondering how the upcoming Sunday would go without me. The church had arranged for one of the deacons or elders to preach. We had learned long ago that there was never a need for an outside guest pastor. We had learned how to take care of each other, how to fill in for each other, how to work with each other. I knew it would all go just fine, and so it did.

When people came by for a visit, I tired almost immediately. Glad as I was to see them, it took all the strength I had to maintain a presence. As all people do after a crisis we soon developed a heart-felt shorthand to convey what happened. "They say I shouldn't be talking at all," I'd say. "They say I really shouldn't have made it, but here I am. I am so thankful. And soon back I'll be." Then the guests would gently leave, overlooking the pronunciation slips, and the dull drone of my robot voice. After they left I would easily drift off to sleep giving thanks for a congregation that reached out to us with exquisite kindness, concern and prayer when my own capacity to live those very same values had seemingly vanished.

Sunday came and went. Monday came and went. I resolved to not say "I'm sorry" or "dang!" or, more often, "there I go again" when I missed a word. One morning Tim and I walked over to church.

"Would you like to hear the Bach?" I asked him. Piano had been one of my sabbatical pursuits, and a gifted piano teacher in Big Timber had allowed it to continue. The first piece of the *Well Tempered Clavichord* is an astoundingly beautiful piece of music in the beginner's key of "C." If theology is the pursuit of harmony, then music is perhaps its closest cousin, as Schopenhauer so astutely pointed out.[t] It is in the arts that we approach the sacred, and restore our soul in an all too often brutal world. The words "minister" and "minstrel" are related for good reason. The banjo was my instrument of choice, but although it had blessings that included making it impossible to play a sad song, it couldn't quite compete with the piano and the etherial harmonies Bach so lovingly and beautifully found for it. Besides, the piano was at church and playing for Tim gave me a reason to enter the sanctuary. Tim said he'd be glad to hear the piece.

I switched on the Kawai digital piano, pushed the "Mellow Grand" button, and gently placed my fingers on the keys. I knew the piece almost by heart, so I was sure I could play it for him. Just to make sure, I leaned the music on its stand, took a deep breathe, and then began to play. After a few measures, the piece disintegrated. The notes no longer told my hands just where to go. The

---

I never knew a thing about Schopenhauer until my strokes. Bryan McGee's note about him, in his book, *The Story of Thought*, DK Publishing, London, 1998, page 144, nearly stopped me in my tracks. "In Schopenhauer's view there is only one way in which we can find momentary release from our imprisonment in the dark dungeon of this work, and that is through the arts. In painting, sculpture, poetry, drama, and above all music, the otherwise relentless rack of willing on which we are stretched out throughout life is relaxed, and suddenly we find ourselves free from the tortures of our existence. For a moment we are in touch with something outside the empirical real, a different order of being: we literally have the experience of being taken out of time and space altogether, and also out of ourselves, even out of the material object that is our body."

synapses that connect a visual note with the strike of a finger, and the tone I imagined in my heart, failed to fire. It was almost dizzying to just look at the notes; and the fact that I couldn't figure it all out brought on frustration.

"Wait a minute, I'll get it. I'll get it."

"Relax, Dad," Tim said, responding to my rising anxiety.

"Geez. Wait a minute. Let me try it again." Once again the notes were a prelude to confusion. My hope to share a piece of music with my firstborn son was out of reach. We put on our jackets and walked back home.

Tuesday came and went.

I got up. Worked out. Put on my jacket and decided to go back over to church. There is something about putting on one's jacket before walking to work that has almost magical powers. It is the first thing we do as we cross the threshold from home to the world and so it takes on almost protective power. The way we dress signals coherence. The white doctor's coat says, "I'm the doctor." The minister's stole says, "I know about God." What we wear ends confusion about who we are and how we are to act. Jackets are the same way. Putting on a jacket and walking out the door meant there was work to be done. When I arrived at church I went into my office and sat down at the computer to send some e-mails, and to see what mail might have come in. I was typing away when Byron came in.

"What are you doing?" he said, "trying to kill yourself?" No human being on earth could say those words with more kindness and concern than Byron Manley. In his late seventies (though I never actually asked him to pin it down), Byron had been a rancher, the town grocer, and a jack of all trades. He was on the pastoral care committee. He never wore his faith on his sleeve. He didn't need to. If it was Sunday, he was there. If an idea needed careful weighing he was part of the conversation. When the nursing home needed an ombudsman, he volunteered. I was glad to see him. Noting that I still didn't have a snap-button western shirt after living in town a few years, he took it on himself to quietly pass one of his my way.

"Oh no," I said, "I'll be okay."

"Well for crying out loud, what are you doing? You had better take it easy."

"Well I'm just trying to catch up on things. I won't be here long."

"I hope not." The gentle but firm chide in his voice spoke of concern. We chatted a bit more, and I recited the litany that had become second nature to me. "I'm lucky I lived. Glad I can *stlock*. No, there I go again. Glad I can *talk*. I'll be okay."

I finished the work nobody had asked me to do and sent an e-mail to Gary Gunderson with whom I'd been collaborating on a book about boundary leadership. We met when I traveled as part of a Montana team to Atlanta for a conference run by the Interfaith Health Program. Our goal was astonishingly simple: we wanted to reform healthcare by remembering that because faith communities and hospital systems both care about healing, they ought to have something to do with each other. At the end of the four day workshop Gary mentioned he was working on a book about people who lived their lives at the very edges of their professions. Boundary leaders are people whose creative spirits won't take "no" for an answer and who know how to push, prod, lead and inspire churches and institutions to live up to their highest hopes. I offered to interview some boundary leaders to put a face on his ideas. Over the next few months I interviewed a Norwegian neurologist, a Dallas pastor, a Los Angeles organizer, a Chicago theologian and several South Africans, asking them each to share the essences of their lives. It was a good partnership and the interviews eventually appeared in his book, *Boundary Leadership*. In my e-mail I told him I'd had a stroke, that the next interview might have to wait a bit but that I was still on track with the project that had inspired both me and the congregation with which I shared what I'd been learning from a new network of friends.

I appreciated Byron's common sense words that lovingly reminded me of the boundary I wanted to explore.

chapter six
aftershocks

• • •

First the earthquake, and then the aftershocks.

I had completed my work out. Twenty minutes aerobic. Half an hour of weights and sit-ups. I went a little harder than normal, wanting to make up for the days of exercise lost in the hospital.

Took a shower. Dried off, dressed, put on a newly pressed orange shirt. Sat down on the edge of my bed feeling a bit faint. There are, of course, a million reasons why a diabetic feels faint.

Closed my eyes.

And that is the last thing I remember.

I was suddenly convulsing in a *grand mal* seizure. My eyes rolled back into my head. My hands, arms and legs all convulsed wildly. Tim was the first to hear me fall. He came running and tried to steady me, making sure I wouldn't hurt myself. Connie came as fast as she could. In a few minutes the seizure subsided. By that time, Casey had bounded into our room and started to lick my face. It turns out that dogs have an uncanny capacity to respond to seizures and there have even been some attempts to train them to spot a seizure before it happens. Connie called 911 and the ambulance crew appeared almost immediately. There was no way to know at that time if the seizure was the harbinger of another stroke. Although I had experienced convulsions from a hypoglycemic reaction in the past, I had never had an epileptic seizure before.

"Seizures are like electrical storms," said David as we talked about that day. "They start when one part of the brain fires, and then another part fires, and pretty soon both hemispheres are firing. It overwhelms the brain and the electrical impulses that control the body lose their capacity to do what they are supposed to do. With the loss of control comes the chaos of a seizure."

"But what caused it in the first place?" I asked.

"It could have been just a bit of scar tissue from the stroke. Scar tissue can act as an irritant. We don't know why it becomes a focal point, but we have found that if we do surgery and take out the scar tissue, the seizures stop.

"And your stroke, like all strokes, made your brain fragile. There is a thing called the 'seizure threshold' that prevents these neural thunderstorms. For most people the threshold is very high, and we never reach it. It's kind of like a ceiling that prevents us from reaching or jumping too high. Because it's there we don't hurt ourselves. But a TBI or stroke lowers the ceiling. So does alcohol, and so does becoming overly fatigued. One way to measure the seizure threshold is to hook a person up to an EEG and then deprive the person of sleep for 24 or 48 hours. That forces a seizure and the threshold level can be recorded. The good news is that, for most people, a seizure in and of itself does not cause damage to the brain. It is not like having another stroke."

I have no memory of being taken to the hospital. I do remember awakening surrounded by all the hospital accouterments: nurses in their light blue uniforms, the large pillows under my head and beside me, the visits by Kirby in his white coat, and Connie's loving presence. I reached out to take her hand, squeezing it, heartened she was there. And I slept. And slept. And slept still more.

From time to time nurses kept asking me to do the same things I'd been asked to do at the hospital in Billings -- pull their arms towards me as they resisted the pull, push against them with both legs, and follow their fingers as they moved them in front of my face. Once again the tests seemed silly. Although I mispronounced an occasional word, fatigue presented itself as the problem and surely a few days of rest would take care of that. The seizure was no more than an aftershock.

Shirts have an odd way of speaking to us. When I was taken to the hospital in Rumford, Maine, for the first days of my life as a diabetic, I wore a bright red shirt. For some 54 years since then, I have consistently avoided red shirts. I know, of course, that the red shirt had nothing to do with my diagnosis, and that associating red shirts with the end of my "regular life" and the beginning of my life as a diabetic is silly. But in the years since I've opted for green, or blue, or white, or orange shirts. Anything but red. On the day of my seizure I wore an orange button up shirt. It was an Izod shirt, to be precise, one we bought in St. Louis when we were on sabbatical. I liked that shirt, its bright color reminded me of the sabbatical experience made up of writing, music and my association with the Interfaith Health Program. For one reason or another we began calling it my "lucky shirt." On the second day in the hospital, I wanted to change from the hospital gown back into my clothes, which had been stashed away in the narrow closet.

I opened the closet door, saw the lucky shirt, and took it off the hanger.

I looked at the buttons, searched the sleeves to see whether or not they were inside out and began to put it on like I had so many times before. But instead of figuring it out I fumbled. The buttons and the buttonholes seemed to belong to utterly separate worlds. My hands were too big to perform such a small sequential task. I couldn't connect all the things I was supposed to do, and was sure I should have known how to do:

> Find the button;
> Match it with the proper hole;
> Check to see if it's the right one;
> Fix it if it isn't.
> Start again from the top if you can't get it.
> No matter what I did I couldn't get it.

Fumbling. Stupid shirt. I was fumbling. And it wasn't just my hands that couldn't figure it out. Neither could my elbow, or arms. Balance betrayed me. I could not get the shirt on, the crumbled shirt that needed ironing. Putting it on became a baffling and complicated puzzle. The lucky shirt had run out of luck. Connie saw me struggling with it, and helped out. I put the nightgown back on, laid down, and, once again, fell asleep, losing track of time.

When I awoke, the large clock on the wall stared straight at me. It was exactly what a clock is supposed to be. It had twelve numbers, and three hands: the hour hand, the minute hand, and the second hand which took 30 seconds to fall, and then 30 seconds to rise on its appointed rounds. I stared at the clock and realized with an almost sickening sensation that I had absolutely no idea what time it was.

"It's a clock, you can tell time," I said to myself. "You know how to tell time. You learned how to do this when you were three years old."

True enough. But truth didn't change the fact that I had no idea how to read the clock. I tried again to decipher the time, working through the strange problem as though it was a college exam. Once again I came up short. A clock is all about relationship. One cannot tell the time if one does not understand the relationship between the short hour hand and the big minute hand, to say nothing of the extra-long second hand. One cannot tell time if one does not understand the time relationship between the number 10 on the dial and the relative position of the clock's two hands. It is the right brain that deciphers relationships. I was staring at the clock but could not tell the time. After three or four minutes the dials finally made sense and the time of day snapped into place. When I later looked at the clock; time once again eluded me. Then it snapped back into place and made sense. Each time I looked at it I knew I'd need time to tell the time.

Three days later, it was finally time to go home. Medically, my brain was still fragile. Kirby prescribed Tegretol, a powerful anti-seizure medication that he said would knock me out, and so it did. Its levels needed constant monitoring. I was also taking Plavix to thin out my blood, aspirin, and an antidepressant. Post-stroke depression is par for the course and prescribing an antidepressant is akin to asking a heart attack survivor to take an aspirin each day. It is an almost automatic procedure. I teasingly told Connie that the only other thing we needed was a new lucky shirt.

"No way," she said. "No lucky shirts for you." Blue might work; or white; or green; but not orange, and red was out of the question.

"There may have been other factors regarding the seizure," David said. "Everything that happens to you is far more complex than it is for normal people because of your diabetes. You can't separate that from whatever happens to you. Things that a normal person could shake off you can't shake off. You've taken good care of yourself and lived with Type 1 for half a century, but you still got hit by the stroke and the seizure. And now with the deficits that came from your stroke, managing your diabetes can't help but be more difficult than ever. You have two, maybe three, worlds to track all the time—diabetes, the stroke, and your heart. Any one of them can throw the other two off course. You've got a lot going on and it makes your overall health precarious."

He was right.

We weren't far away from Thanksgiving, and in 2003 the town's service would be held at our church. I realize that doesn't sound like much if you live in Chicago or Boston, but it had been six or seven years since we were chosen to host and I was determined it would be the best service ever. For a number of years attendance at the services had been sparse, so we wanted to find a way to turn that around. Long before November 11 we began to "line out," as we say in Montana, the music, the youth group's part of the service, the scripture readings, the refreshments and the offerings. We had put up signs in the front windows of stores up and down McLeod Avenue. Just as we supported the stores, they supported us, always saying, "Go right ahead, and post whatever you'd like." I rarely shopped at stores that did not allow their windows to become community bulletin boards. In general, the larger the store, the less likely it was.

I was bound and determined to do the service. Everyone had been so kind, so concerned; I owed them something. Were it up to me I would be there if it was the last thing I did. But thankfully it was not up to me.

chapter seven
rules

...

It is an odd thing to perceive but not understand. Perception alone is a matter of the five senses: sight, touch, smell, sound and taste. The sixth sense is often considered to be intuitive understanding. That may well be the case but I have come to believe the sixth sense is thought. The five senses guide us along the road of perception, but they must be wrapped in thought to yield understanding. When we take away relational thinking, and can see a clock but not read its time, we find ourselves in a void and have no idea how to find the door. It is more bewildering than frightening, more ethereal than bewitching. Remove thought from perception and the earth is as empty and void as it was before God separated night from day.

I had sensed when I looked into Floyd's eyes that there was far more going on in his mind than he could say, when I asked him, "What's it like?" As my brain began to settle down from both the seizure and the stroke, I tried to answer the question in the realm of everyday experience. I awoke each morning, did my workout, drank a cup of coffee, turned on Morning Edition and sat down with *The Billings Gazette*. It had never been difficult to read the paper and listen to the radio at the same time. In fact, it was an immensely pleasurable experience. Give me a newspaper, any newspaper, and I'm happy. I had always loved the saying that a pastor should never fail to carry the Bible under one arm and the newspaper under the other.

But things had changed. The radio was now a distraction. To make sense of the paper and comprehend the radio, while seemingly simple, required multitasking. I would turn the radio down and read the paper without its interference. Despite the best work of reporters and editors, sentence after sentence failed to convey the intended meaning. There had to be meaning in those words, but nothing registered. I would read a sentence again, pronouncing each word out loud in my thoughts. Sometimes, on the third or fourth try, the words and their meanings fell into place, but at other times the sentence still made no sense. At first I thought it had to be the writer's fault. "Who on earth wrote that sentence? That's the worst sentence I've ever read in my life!" I would say to myself. But although perhaps they could have been better, the sentences weren't the problem. And neither was the clock. The words and the numbers were doing exactly what words and numbers do--conveying meaning. Ferreting out that meaning was an unwelcome exercise in damage assessment.

These memories form but half the picture. It took others to reveal what I did not, and could not, know. Connie could tell that I was hearing, but not understanding, much of what she and Kirby said. How reassuring it would have been to have attributed the loss of communication to the normal causes — the normal distances that separate husbands from their wives, and wives from their husbands or patients from the counsel of their physicians. One does not need to have a stroke or a traumatic brain injury to cause a failure to communicate. In some ways a stroke simply accentuates already existing *cul de sacs* in any relationship. Whereas I tended to see the big picture, she focused on details I preferred to avoid. When I ran into difficulties with one of my earlier congregations, it almost broke her trust in the word "church." For me, church was always a source of hope, no matter how many difficulties we experienced. Whereas I tended to be social, she tended to keep to herself both by nature and the disability that hemmed her life on so many fronts. When I misperceived reality, she would gently, but persistently, point it out to me.

"Don't you remember?" she would ask.

"No."

"We've already talked about that."

"We did? I never heard that."

"Yes, we did."

Throughout it all, she was far more aware of my disabilities than I was. Her connection to "reality" was not always welcome, but was, and is, always essential.

As I tried to hold on to some semblance of reality, it seemed as though there was not room in my brain to both do what I was doing and to respond to her. "His brain is full," Kirby once said to her. "And you can't get in." His words were unsettlingly true. Perhaps if I had stopped trying to get better there would have been more room for the give and take relationship we had shared throughout our marriage. The grocery store---too much. Reading the paper and listening to the radio--too much. Making sense of poorly written sentences--too much. We seemed to be living out the words God gave to the prophet Isaiah: "You may listen and listen, but you will not understand. You may look and look again, but you will never know [so that] you may turn and be healed." (Isaiah 6:9). Healing belonged to a world we could hope for but not quite touch.

It is tempting to attribute lapses of communication to the realm of psychology. The urge to remain in control, even when wrong; the heroic if misinformed, need to overcome any obstacle; and the friction that characterizes any marriage are all part of the human condition. The presence of brain damage merely accentuates what is already in play in any relationship. It is often reported that traumatic brain injury, whether from a stroke or an accident, foreshadows divorce. The observation is used to impress the listener, making it appear that the trauma was so severe that no marriage in the world could survive such a situation. And, there certainly are times when trauma does indeed jeopardize or even end marriages. But it turns out that statistics do not bear out armchair psychology. It is not true that the change in patterns of communication automatically lead to separation or divorce. When life has lost its coherence, and chaos seems to roar on all sides, it is the world of vows that gives us hope. We had said, "for better or worse," "in sickness and in health" not knowing what the future held. In the ensuing years life made sure we came to realize the depth of the vows we shared as disability increasingly came our way.

"Guess what?" I would always say to couples who stood before the church to share their marriage vows.

"You have absolutely no idea what lays ahead."

They and the church would laugh.

"But this one thing you know. Whatever it is, you have vowed to share it together. Such is the nature of marriage."

Connie sensed the danger I could not fully grasp. I had been sneaking over to church to try and regain a sense of place. My robe with its stoles was on its hanger in my office, beneath the placard Connie gave me that read, *Pobody's Nerfect*. The symbols of my life were in that room and I wanted to be in their presence. Finally Connie called Kirby and asked to see him. She tells the story this way:

"I went over to their house one night, and said, 'Look I am desperate.' I sat down on their couch beside Julie. Kirby got out a glass of coke, poured some whiskey in it and said, 'What's going on?' He was as great as a person could be. I was still having trouble trying to explain that I wasn't complaining about you, but I was really concerned that there were some dangers I just couldn't get you to see. I was supposed to be the compliance officer on life and death issues, but it was as though you had no idea what we were talking about. It wasn't psychological, it was neurological. I finally realized it might help if I took myself out of the picture a bit. I asked Kirby if he would write down an explicit list of instructions. If the list came from him you might listen because you still respected authority. I asked him to write down the top eight or nine things in plain and simple language. I thought there was a chance the list might implant itself in your mind. It needed to say, 'Don't do this, and don 't do that.' Then we could keep it in plain sight by putting it on the door of the refrigerator.

"He said, 'My God that's brilliant. The only way to help him hear some of this is through some simple statements that don't come from you. If the directions come from you that turns it into a relationship issue, and turns you into his keeper. That's both difficult and humiliating.' He wrote it out right then. When I read it over I started sobbing. Then he signed it and I came home."

I had no idea they had met when Kirby came over the next afternoon. I sat on the couch, Connie beside me, and Kirby in the red chair I had bought to ease the pain in Connie's feet some years before. We chatted a bit, circling before coming to the point. There have been times I've made fun of small talk, and pointed out how ineffectual it is to comment on the weather. But actually ministry is the art of entertaining small talk, knowing there is always something else waiting to surface. If it is cornered too quickly it is likely to disappear. And so we learn to read inflection, to see how a smile fits with the words, or how the words about the weather disguise the emotions that speak of storms on an otherwise sunny day. It is fitting that the word for "wind" and "spirit" are the same in both Greek and Hebrew so perhaps talking about the ever-present Big Timber wind couldn't help but be a spiritual conversation in one way or another. Kirby, Connie and I circled a bit, as people do when first sitting down together. The time came for the small talk to end. I seized the moment and leaned forward a bit.

"Is the Thanksgiving service really out?" I asked.

"It's out," he said. He said that the service would be just fine without my presence; that my sermon could be read; that my doing it would be unwise, to say the least. It wouldn't take much to provoke yet another aftershock. Besides, it would be embarrassing for me to get up there and make a fool of myself in ways I could not foresee. There were two streams of thought in his counsel. One aimed at preventing another seizure or stroke. The second was intended to help set the stage for a new life. To do that I'd have to let go of the old one. I nodded my head. It was a sermon I had given almost every Sunday of my life: let go of the old, embrace the new, and trust that God would stay with us through it all. But he could see by the look on my face that I was determined to hold on to the reins. His words didn't phase me. The cells responsible for comprehending the import of such a message no longer existed.

A new word began to creep into the conversation: *Anosognosia*. One book defines it as "the devastating condition that strips the patient of the capacity for insight into his own illness. A patient with anosognosia may be severely impaired, yet he will have no inkling of it and will continue to claim that everything is fine. This is different from being 'in denial,' when it is assumed that the patient has the capacity to comprehend his own deficit but chooses to look the other way. Following frontal lobe damage the cognitive capacity for insight into one's own condition is genuinely lost." Connie and Kirby were not vying against a stubborn husband and a noncompliant patient. They were up against anosognosia.

It was time for boundaries. Kirby handed me a lined piece of paper entitled "The Rules of the Road to Healing". The letters were large, the handwriting clear.

The Rules of the Road to Healing

1. You will not preach at the Thanksgiving service.
2. You need to remain in controlled situations with only one or two people in the room at the same time.
3. All communications, such as letters, must first be cleared with me or Connie. There will be no exceptions to this.
4. You must stay away from the piano or your banjo at this time. This is a must.
5. You may not walk downtown alone.
6. You must not go over to the church or think of returning to work for three months.
7. You may read for a span of 20 minutes, but no longer.
8. Because of the severity of your stroke, you must not provide counseling to people from the church or community.

There will be no exceptions to these rules. I share them with you not because I want to, but because they are essential if you are to continue with your life. I share them because I love you, and respect you, and these are your best chance for healing.

It was relational medicine at its very best. As I write these words I am humbled at the depth of concern he and Connie so lovingly crafted into a safety net. I was touched and appreciative, and respected the authoritative words. I wish I could write that I took them to heart. Instead, I nodded my head and began to negotiate. If not Thanksgiving, surely the Christmas Eve service would be possible?

"No," he said. "Christmas Eve is out of the question. You do not want to stand up there and be overwhelmed, missing words, unaware of what you're saying or what's going on. No. I can't, and won't, let you do Christmas Eve. It's way too risky."

"But it's a month away. What if I get better?"

"No," he said. "Out of the question."

I nodded, and as I did the age-old scripts kicked in. Each one told the same story: the impossible is possible. When there's a will there's a way. Can't never could. The lepers are healed; the blind see; the crippled walk once again; Helen Keller speaks; a man with no legs climbs Everest, a child awakes from a coma; even death is not the final word. There must be a way to overcome disease.

When I was a child our family put on a yearly production of Gian Carlo Menotti's opera *Amahl and the Night Visitors*. We built a stage, made string marionettes out of *papier mache*, sewed the costumes, tape-recorded the opera, and invited the entire neighborhood for the Christmas production and gave the proceeds to the American Diabetes Association.

The gist of the opera involves a heroic and successful struggle to overcome disability. The three kings are on their way to Bethlehem laden with gifts for the Christ child. They pass through a small village and ask if they might spend a night in one of its homes. Amahl's mother welcomes them into her sparse home and we soon see that her son, Amahl, cannot walk without a crutch. He would like to travel with the kings, but it is out of the question. A crippled boy could never make such a trip. As the kings describe the sumptuous gifts they brought for the Christ child, Amahl's mother is overtaken by temptation. If she took just a few coins perhaps she could afford a cure. Surely the kings would never miss it. After the kings fall asleep, she quietly reaches for a coin, singing softly, "For my child, for my child, for my child." The kings awake and catch her red-handed.

"Thief!" one of the kings sings with a loud and angry voice that virtually takes the breath away from an audience that dared not make a sound as she reached for the gold. Amahl quickly comes to his mother's defense. She poignantly explains that she had waited her entire life for an opportunity to help her child.

Her words melt the kings' anger. Deeply moved, they put aside their anger and eloquently note that the Christ child has no need of gold, that his kingdom will not be one of riches or gold. The depth of their witness prompts Amahl to realize he, too, would like to give a gift, but has only one gift to give -- his crutch. Haltingly, he holds it out and takes a step, and then another, and then another. "He walks," sings one of the kings in a sonorous bass voice. "He walks," sings the baritone. "He walks," sings the gleeful tenor. "He walks," they all sing and soon Amahl joins them, singing in tones only a boy soprano can touch, "Look Mother, I can walk, I can dance, I can run!"

Disease and disability had met their match. The purpose of life is not to protect self, the purpose is to give self away. Such a purpose inevitably contradicts well-meaning advice and scientifically correct medical advice. It was not prudent for Amahl to take that first step or to even dream he might accompany the kings. The rules were prudent, and Connie's intervention was intended to bless whatever healings there might be. But, perhaps, just perhaps, by Christmas I'd be strong enough, to lead a procession of life and light.

The road to acceptance is never a singular path. It has its detours. Denial eventually leads to anger; anger proves fruitless and yields to will-power, which is never strong enough to transcend disease. Will-power is replaced by magical thinking, which would transfer Amahl's magical moment into the lives of every crippled child. Magical thinking yields to a crisis, and the crisis leads to a deeper understanding of surrender. Each detour has its reasons as we all try to control the chaos of disease. It is not surprising that we do this. After all, when Pandora opened the chest, disease was one of the enemies that escaped to torment the world. It is in league with war, famine, despair and evil. Each of them deserves resistance. It is no wonder we ferociously cling to life and do all we can to resist the restraints of disease.

"Is Christmas a possibility?"

"No."

He had to be wrong. There had to be a way. Once again fatigue wrapped me in its weary arms.

Sunday services posed a dilemma. The church, of course, knew exactly what to do. When I left for sabbatical in January, 2003, we organized the church into 12 "Care Neighbor" groups and assigned each group a Sunday. They would do Bible study together, choose the hymns, bring in whatever displays they wanted, and select one person to give the sermon. The plan worked exceedingly well, and when I returned people were on cloud nine. "You should have seen how well we did," many of them said. Now that I was out of action they would simply reassign the groups for a while. Because attending church would break the rule concerning controlled situations, Sunday mornings turned into a different kind of Sabbath. How odd it was to be out of place, to be away from the congregation of people whose lives had become my life. Prayer was still out of reach. The world of "God" felt empty and far away. Breakfasts were hit or miss. Everything, with the exception of hot spices, tasted strangely metallic: metallic oatmeal, metallic fruit, metallic toast. Eating was no fun and without the incentive of taste, I just stopped eating, or ate very little. Needless to say, I began losing weight. Sundays passed. Friends stopped by, though they too received the word that visits were to be limited. Mondays came and went; Tuesdays came and went; each day a workout, each day a hope, each day a collapse, each day an expectation that something might happen, each day bringing us one step closer to Christmas, and one step closer to a better understanding of what happened when the leaves fell on that fall day.

In a time of medical crisis, specialists reign supreme. We give them extraordinary power. We expect that years of training will enable them to easily separate the wheat from the chaff. As the children's disabilities increased, and as Connie's condition deteriorated, we turned to the famed Mayo Clinic and Shriners' Hospital for Crippled Children assured that we would be in the hands of "one of the best." Such expectations eclipse the healing power of a primary care physician, and lead us to expect a cure is just around the corner. In our case we wondered if a consultation with a neurologist might shed light on what had happened and what the prognosis for healing might be. Kirby took care to consult with a number of them about my case, and found one he thought would be a good fit.

We scheduled the appointment and anxiously waited for the day to arrive. We had told all the stories there were to tell. The holding pattern begged for new information to break its spell. When the day came we drove to Billings, and entered the vast medical complex. It is amazing how many portals one must pass through before arriving at a specialist's office.

By the time one arrives in the concentrated space of a small exam room, the appointment is important and expensive, and perhaps even powerful enough and expensive enough to provide a cure. After all those transitions one is surprised to find there are yet a few more steps.

"Mr. Pray?" the receptionist called. We went forward and a nurse led us down a short hallway to a small room. The doctor wasn't there, but I looked at the degrees and certificates on her wall, one of which certified that she had climbed Mount Kilimanjaro. That was impressive. I had once hiked in the hills and valleys of South Africa's Drakensburgs, finding them, as Alan Paton wrote, "lovely beyond any singing of it." To hike in Africa is an unforgettable experience. No wonder she kept that certificate on her wall. We shared something in common. Perhaps that was a good omen. Kirby trusted her, and had filled her in on the rules of healing and the troubling collision between compliance and the perception. She understood she would need to be direct, that her words might not strike home, that she would have to find ways to demonstrate the toll the stroke had taken. As the Chinese proverb puts it, "I hear and I forget; I see and I remember; I do and I understand."

We waited.

For some reason I did not want to sit down. I don't know why. I do know that in the months following the stroke, that same reluctance stayed with me. The doctor finally came into the room; sat down; and then asked me to sit down. Then she performed a few of the same tests they had conducted in the hospital a few weeks earlier. I followed the tips of her fingers with my eyes as they moved far to the left; then to the right. She seemed surprised my vision was clear, that my eyes had no problem simultaneously tracking her fingers. She asked me to push against her palm with my right arm; then my left arm. And then she took out a pin.

At first she gently pricked the right side of my skull in five or six places, asking me if I could feel anything.

"Yes," I said. It felt exactly the way it was supposed to feel. Then she moved to the left side of my head. But this time I couldn't feel the pressure. I knew I should feel something, but I didn't. The difference between the two sides amazed me. She went back and again pricked the left side of my skull.

"Feel that?"

"No, not really," I said. "It's dull."

"Let's try your feet." I took off my socks and sat on the edge of the examining table.

"Can you feel that?" she asked as she pushed the dull pin against the bottom of my right foot.

"Yes."

"Good." I was proud of that feeling. Fifty years of diabetes has a way of erasing feeling from the bottom of one's foot, but I'd always been able to feel a pin or a feather brushed against the bottom of my feet. It always felt like a victory against the odds. I could outrun anything that was supposed to come after me. Then she took the pin to my left foot.

"Can you feel that?"

"No. Not really." Again I couldn't believe the difference. I could see her pressing the pin, but it only felt dull, or didn't really "feel" at all.

"Can you feel that?"

"No. That's weird. I didn't feel that."

"Okay," she said.

I was once again shocked at the difference between my right and my left side. Her simple tests were revealing something that had eluded my attention. The left side of my body had lost part of its capacity to feel.

"Have you seen your MRI?" she asked.

"No," we answered.

"Well, lets go look at it and I'll show you why you're not feeling things on the left side of your body. Come with me." We followed her as she left the exam room, leading us into another room with a wall designed for viewing X-rays. She took the large black film out of its packet, switched on a panel of lights behind a plastic case, and pushed the MRI under its clips. It's odd how doctors have different ways of doing that. Some throw the films up against the screen with such upward force that they automatically slip under the clips. Some begin their perusal of the film in the room's ambient light and then carefully place them up against the brightly lit screen to confirm their original hunch. Only then do they

tend to pay attention to the patient and begin to share the story of what the films reveal and the future holds.

She carefully secured the film under the clips and stepped to the side. We moved forward. It is always strange to look at one's skull. The jaw seems huge, the eye sockets loom like craters of the moon, the cranium appears as a misshaped planet that lost its center of gravity. My skull looked exactly like the skull Yorik held as Hamlet and Horatio came walking by, or the skulls found in the killing fields of Cambodia or in the trenches of some archaeological dig. But MRIs show more than the skull; they also show tissue inside the skull. It was the tissue that caught our eye and stole our breath. A cloud of anguished astonishment crossed Connie's face. I could hear the breath leave her. She said nothing. She could say nothing. Neither could I as we let the pictures sink into our lives. The left side was uniformly gray, with darker grays here and there, just the way it was supposed to be. The pictures of brains I'd seen in the anatomy book made it clear that white tissue was a problem. Live brain cells show up gray; dead cells show up white. For the most part, the right side of my brain was white. It looked like Antarctica had untethered herself and drifted into my brain. It wasn't a small area, or one or two places that were white –the entire right side of my brain looked like a lost continent.

"That's where the stroke happened," the doctor said. "All of those cells are dead." Her words were monosyllabic, each punctuated with the emphasis only a single syllable can give. All...of...those...cells...are...dead.

I reached out for Connie's hand. Neither of us could believe what we saw. Now, for a moment, we could understand why the nurses had said it was a miracle I had survived. Billions of nerve cells had simply drowned, just as surely as leaves had fallen from the maple at the corner of Fifth and McLeod. Once gone, they were gone, and would not come to life again.

I stepped back to the exam bed, and leaned up against it.

"Okay," I said. "What do I do?" My voice may have been monotone but its intent was unmistakable. The specialist surely had a way to undo what had happened. I felt much the same way I had when I learned I'd be taking insulin for the rest of my life. "Okay," I'd said, "I can live with that." After all life goes on. Let's engage this battle. Tell me what to do and I'll do it. I was ready for whatever instruction the doctor and MRI had to give. She looked at me, sensing both what I was saying and deeply aware of what I didn't understand.

"You don't understand. Those cells are gone," she said. Connie remembers her voice as a mixture of kindness and firm truth. I don't remember her voice that way at all. I remember her speaking with grim certainty that would not allow any sidestepping of the neurological truth. To me her words were the work of the grim reaper. "They don't grow back. They're dead. Nerve cells don't regenerate."

I took a deep breath. I'm sure Connie did as well. We could scarcely believe what she had said as the MRI continued to stare at us from the illuminated wall.

"Okay," I said again. "What do we do?"

"You must not work for at least three months," she said. Three months. I could live with that. It wasn't what the king had said, but I could live with that. The seizure let me know things were fragile. And I was so tired so much of the time, the rest would be a blessing. Then she drew a set of boundaries, just as Kirby had done. Whereas Kirby's came wrapped in compassion, the neurologist had no such leaning. Her sentences were short, her words terse. I was a problem, not a patient.

"Do you drink coffee?"

"Yes."

"Not anymore."

"Do you drink alcohol?"

"Yes," I said. I almost inserted the "proven" fact that a glass or two of red wine is healthy for the heart. But this wasn't a time for commentary.

"Not anymore."

She moved to diabetes.

"Do you know what to do if your blood sugar is low?"

"Of course. I take some juice or something sweet."

"No," she said. "You have to take glucose tablets. You cannot afford to have a low blood sugar and it has been shown that glucose tablets are the best and fastest way out of a reaction." I didn't ask her why low blood sugars were more dangerous now than they had been.

"Will I eventually be able to return to work?" I asked.

"It's doubtful," she said. Once again Connie and I had a sinking feeling.

"So what do we do now?" I asked. I felt like a boy scout asking for instructions that would earn me a merit badge. I was not going to do nothing.

"You're going to need therapy," she said. "I think New Hope would be the best place." Billings, Montana, like so many other cities, has two hospitals on what's come to be known as the city's medical campus. Both of them trace their roots to the goodwill of churches. The Methodists founded Deaconess Hospital, which later merged with the Billings Clinic, which markets itself as the Mayo Clinic of the Northwest. The other, St. Vincent Healthcare, was founded by the Sisters of Charity of Fort Leavenworth, Kansas, whose mission it was to provide healthcare to the poor. Most of my care, for one reason or the other, was at Deaconess, and that's where my neurologist had her office. But it didn't have a therapeutic ward for inpatient stroke or TBI victims. St. Vincent's however, did specialize in rehabilitation, designating an entire hospital floor for traumatic brain injury and stroke patients. They called the unit New Hope.

"How do we go about contacting them?"

"I've already done that," she said. "Just go up there."

" Now?"

"Yes."

The appointment was over. It was the last time I would ever see her.

We thanked her for the visit, took the heavy MRI films, pushed them back into their manila packets, and headed out for the car. Connie drove the four blocks north to St. Vincent's. Although I had been there many times visiting parishioners, I couldn't remember where the New Hope floor was. St. Vincent's is a melange of buildings and navigation is anything but easy. Staff are actually trained to spot confusion on visitors' faces and then help them find the appropriate elevator. We looked at the signs, found an elevator, and went up to the fourth floor. Once there we weren't sure where to turn. I knew the walking was painful for Connie. There were wheelchairs she could have used but she would not take advantage of them, just as I would do everything I could to not be a problem for other people. A nurse saw the quizzical expressions on our faces and pointed us in the right direction.

We walked to the New Hope desk. Three or four nurses stood at the desk, all going about their various duties. We waited for a moment, and then one asked if she could help us.

"Yes," I said. "We were sent here by my neurologist. She said I'm supposed to be a patient here." We could tell instantly she had no idea what I was talking about. I was proud I hadn't mispronounced a single word.

"What is your name?"

"Larry Pray, and this is my wife Connie." Once again, a look of confusion. It is astounding how difficult it can be for two separate hospital systems in the same town to coordinate care. Perhaps it is a matter of competition, perhaps hospitals require the doctors from other hospitals to have a special certification before recommendations can be considered. We do not know. We do know that the "yours" and "ours" dynamic is the last thing patients need in times of crisis. With the MRI images fresh in our minds we needed all the help we could get.

"Is this New Hope?"

"Yes."

"We were just told by our neurologist to come here. She said it is all set up." They did not respond. We waited for someone to say, "Oh yes, I took that call. We've been waiting for you." The nurses looked at each other with quizzical expressions and looked over the desk for some telling piece of paper that might end the confusion. No such note appeared.

We stepped back a bit and looked up and down the hallway. Several patients and their nurses were slowly moving in and out of their rooms with the aid of walkers or wheelchairs. Suddenly the problem came into view. I had walked to the desk without assistance. Both of my arms moved. My speech was coherent, with nothing but the drone voice to indicate the lifeless white continent we had just seen. New Hope was for acute patients. Even if the neurologist thought New Hope was exactly where I should be, by all outward appearances I didn't belong there. We stood at the desk wondering what to do, where to go and with whom we might speak. It was too late to call the neurologist. We didn't want to call Kirby, as this referral wasn't his.

"There must have been a mix-up," I said. "I'm sorry." We stepped back from the desk and walked back to the elevator, stunned by what happened, and still trying to come to terms with the scope of the damage the MRI had revealed. Hope evaporated. A place for recovery evaporated; the hope for recovery was "doubtful," the route ahead of us was uncertain. The hope-filled stories we anticipated sharing with friends and the church could not find their words.

With the possible exception of March, all months are beautiful. The dark sky of a December night allows the stars to shine with stunning clarity. The snow bounces light back to the heavens; the ice heaves on the banks of the Yellowstone River are a kaleidoscope of gray, white, light green, and pale blues that change shape and color with each new freeze. When life crashes, and prayer loses its power of appeal, one turns to creation. Perhaps we cannot speak with God, but on all sides creation surrounds us with eloquence. The wandering river is God's river, so is the deep darkness of the night sky, the canopy of stars, the snow and fields whose grasses pierce their frozen crust. Sixty miles west of Billings, the Crazy Mountains appear with the great plains sweeping up to their foothills.

It is not surprising that when words lose power, music makes up for the loss. If all we knew about faith is what we find in the hymnal of any denomination, it would be enough. As Isaac Watts wrote in 1775,

> I sing the mighty power of God that made the mountains rise,
> That spread the flowing seas abroad and built the lofty skies.
> I sing the wisdom that ordained the sun to rule the day;
> The moon shines full at God's command, and all the stars obey.

Such sentiments carried us as we returned home.

But so did anger born of both understandings and misunderstandings that had contradicted themselves all day long. We later learned that the neurologist had not realized ambulatory patients were not eligible for New Hope's services and was aghast at what happened after we left her office. Taken together, the day's events were devoid of hope. Pure emotion surfaced as we reacted to the specialist who said, "those cells are gone" but had no magic potion to bring them back. The fallen leaves would have to stay on the ground. We had seen the lost continent and could not find a compass.

When our children were little they learned, as all kids do, that a bad day at work would spill over into their lives in ways they did not deserve. In time they developed a tag for those moments when anger erupted. "That's displaced aggression, Dad," they'd say. And, of course, they were right. Our despair was nothing more than displaced aggression. Thank God for the voice of creation in the midst of despair. Although we may be checkmated, "The heavens are telling the glory of God, and the firmament proclaims his handiwork, their voice goes out through all the earth," just as the ancient hymn of Psalm 19 said it would.

Casey and a warm house welcomed us home.

The day was done.

A new day awaited.

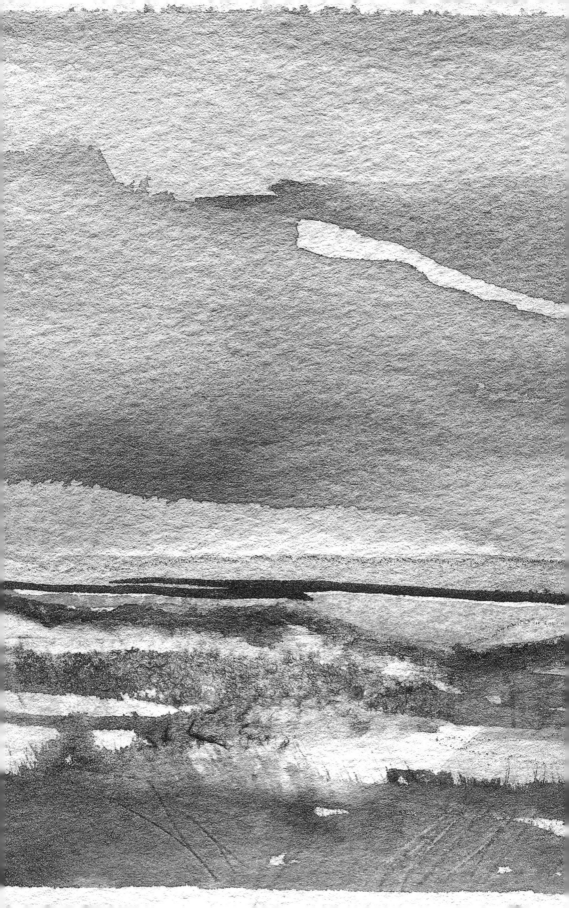

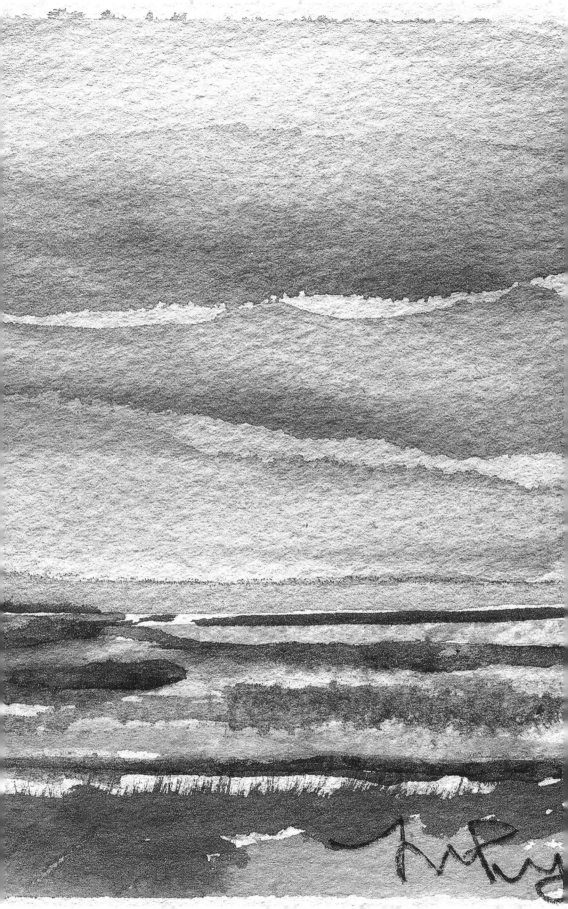

chapter eight
friendship's harmony

• • •

We had stories to tell.

So did Christmas. In the depth of winter its music filled the sky. Each hymn, each carol, wrapped us in the mantle of hope. It may have been the midnight of our lives but the carols spoke of peace that came upon a midnight clear; of angels whose *Gloria, in excelsis, Deo* declared a new connection between God and humankind. Sometimes the music, sometimes the Christmas lights, sometimes the words of carols, sometimes the visits of friends, gently reminded us that much worse could have happened. Life's music could have stopped on November 11 but it did not. Instead the church choir, which had been heeding instructions to gently stay away from our house lest another stroke or seizure occur, came by our porch to share their joyful presence. They could not deny what had happened but would not be overcome by it. Surrounded by song, it was only natural that one morning I tried to sing along with carols brought by choirs or the radio. I am not a good singer but I do love singing and have always been grateful for the perception of the Russian Orthodox Church that the human voice is the only instrument given by God. We made guitars, invented banjos in a burst of genius, figured out how to turn harps into pianos, and learned to turn brass into French Horns and silver into flutes. But these are all human inventions. God gave each of us but one instrument — the human voice. All pastors encourage their congregations to sing without embarrassed restraint. I was never shy about offering that encouragement by singing as best I could from the pulpit. The children, and Connie, tried without success to remind me to turn the microphone off before I began singing. They were right, but I couldn't resist going at music full tilt hoping that if I wasn't afraid to sing the congregation might follow suit.

And so, one morning I tried to sing along with a familiar carol on the radio. With the tune in mind I formed the sound I had always known as singing. But the sound that came out had nothing to do with singing. It sounded like a groan, or an awkward moan. I tried again, and again there was no "voice" to the sound that emerged from my lips. The drone that characterized my spoken voice had extended into the part of the brain responsible for music as well. Rhythm, the capacity to match a note or sing a phrase, to say nothing of a harmony, had all but disappeared and left an awkward and frightening void. Perhaps the deepest compliment we can give to another person is to say, "You've really found your voice." It is in the concept of voice that we harness the gifts of insight, expression, coherence and even the spiritual awareness of call.

I was embarrassed and ashamed that no matter how hard I tried, singing even a single note was impossible. The piano and my beloved banjo were sequestered and the singing proved impossible. Connie called Judy Fjell[7] and asked for help. Judy is a professional musician whose classes, performances and recordings are sources of extraordinary joy. When she is with kids, they sing; when shy adults are in her presence, they suddenly find they can sing. When ten year-old kids learn to play the guitar from her, they find a presence, poise, and confidence that can only come from a gifted teacher and the ethereal power of music. For Judy, music is life, and life is music. When Connie explained to her the stroke had vitually erased my capacity to embrace music, Judy immediately understood how deep such a loss could be. Connie asked her if she might come over to see if we could recover the gift of singing. After all, it might be a form of therapy. Judy said she would find time amid her many classes and recording sessions.

When she came on a snowy day she had her autoharp in hand.

"We're going to start with this," she said.

"Great," I said. I put the harp on my lap, placed one hand over its keypad and the other hand over the strings. It is not a difficult instrument. You push down on the key marked "C" and when you strum a "C"" chord emerges. Push down on

7 For more about Judy's gift of music, go to Judyfjell.com.

the "G" key and a "G" chord emerges. In the hands of a professional the simple instrument can soar. The sounds I made were anything but soaring, but no matter.We were making music.

I suggested to her that we try a song I'd learned from the Quaker hymnal. It had been on my mind for some time, its tune was simple, its words profound. "Cause me to come to thy river, O Lord, cause me to come, cause me to drink, cause me to live." I loved it because it was so true. Often life must cause us to come to the river because left to ourselves we are easily distracted. Then, once there, we might just look at it instead of partaking of its life-giving water. And then, we might just take a sip and head home instead of staying to live by the river. The song was a sermon, the melody and its harmonies were simple and clear. I thought it might be a good song to try.

"Cause me to come to thy river, O Lord," was the first line. I strummed a chord, heard the first note in my mind, and then tried to sing. But once again voice departed me. The sound was embarrassing. I tried again. Once again an utterly atonal sound, midway between a moan and a groan, emerged and any semblance of harmony disappeared. That voice wasn't mine and the sound it made belonged to no one. Judy immediately recognized that the song I'd chosen was too difficult, that I had learned it too recently for it to be embedded in the core regions of my brain. She sensed that only deeply embedded songs might have a chance of harnessing voice.

"Let's work on a song you sang when you were a child," she said.

"Okay."

"How about Go Tell Aunt Rhody?"

"That'll work." It was one of the first songs I'd learned to play on my banjo some 40 years earlier. That should be easy, I thought. She sang the starting note with her clear and compelling voice. I tried to sing the same note and missed it hook, line, and sinker. We tried again. I missed again. We tried again, and this time I found the first note but then had no idea how to tonally move from the "Go tell" to "Aunt" and then on down to "Rhody." She saw the problem and had an idea.

"Here," she said, "follow my hand." Watching her hand move up and down might be another way to access the sounds I could not make. She made one signal for "Go," the same signal for "Tell," then, dropping her hand a bit, another for "Aunt" and, dropping it yet again, another one for "Rhody." I understood the signals but could not connect them with my voice. I was not embarrassed. I was ashamed. After 15 minutes, exhaustion began to rear its ugly head. She could sense my shame, frustration and fatigue. "You were not in good shape," she later said. She had seen through the front I tried so hard to put up. Fortunately, music would not allow such an escape. We thanked her, she left the autoharp, she opened the door and stepped outside into seven or eight inches of snow. I looked over at Connie who could see both despair and fatigue crossing my face. I went upstairs, laid down and once again let sleep try to reclaim the day.

My parents, both in their mid-eighties, flew to Billings from Madison, Wisconsin, to see us. Their presence-sustaining assurance, as we and the children traveled down the roads of chronic disability, had always brought reassurance and safety. It was my mother's arrival in Maine that prompted a visit to the physician who diagnosed diabetes, who took me to the hospital, and who sat beside me in the sunlight patching together a quilt as the first doses of insulin accomplished their miraculous life-giving mission. It was my folks who provided the stability and assurance diabetes required — the regular meals, the rolls of Lifesavers in the car's glove compartment just in case a reaction struck, the trips to the drug store that secured the life-giving vials of insulin. With them disability never trumped life. I'd be just fine traveling to Europe alone, just fine climbing in the Rockies, just fine leaving home and striking out on my own. Their post-stroke presence brought the blessings of home. My dad, ever the scientist, settled down with two books Connie bought to decipher the riddles of brain injury. My mother wanted to meet the many people who had so lovingly surrounded us. Ever the Quaker she held them "in the light." We shared meals together, told a thousand stories, and realized again that although disabilities have the power to alter our lives they do not easily take it away. One way of life had ended; another way of life would surely emerge.

A few weeks after the stroke my mother sent a handwritten note carrying the thoughts of Isaiah Pennington, that eloquently reflected Quaker thought in a time of crisis.

Give over thine own willing,

give over thine own running,

give over thine own desiring to know or be anything

and sink down to the seed which God has sown in thy heart,

and let that be in thee,

and grow in thee,

and breathe in thee,

and act in thee,

and thou shalt find by sweet experience

that God knows that,

and loves that,

and owns that,

and will lead it to the inheritance of life.

We framed the words in a small green frame, that remains on the wall of our apartment to this day. They were true; they had to be true. But I could not protect the tender gift from the real world in which life hit the wall time and time again. As Karl Marx once pointed out, the beauty of the lilies cannot stop a combine of their own accord. I may have been grounded in hope but I still hit the wall. Most survivors of strokes and Traumatic Brain Injury know all about the wall. It's the point where their best effort fails, where our brains seem to short circuit and where it seems like every cell in our body collapses. One afternoon the four of us took a drive into the mountains. Just as they had on our return from the hospital, the telephone poles, and even the fence posts virtually assaulted my vision. One…bam…two…here it comes…three…hit…four…here it comes…another. A regular drive turned into a roller coaster experience. I finally said I was so sorry, but I just had to return home. We drew our expedition to a close and returned home where once again I collapsed.

My mother wanted to meet Cassandra, a member of our church who had taken it upon herself to communicate with everyone on the church e-mail list. Her updates were ever so helpful to both of us. "Larry doesn't quite know how to relate to people," she shared with a congregation wondering what had happened to their pastor and what could be done about it. We invited her over to breakfast one morning along with one other friend. There we were, all six of us, gathered around the breakfast table. It takes breaking down a conversation to see how intricate conversation actually is, how many interchanges there are, how many sounds exist around a table, how much tracking there is as one conversation slides into another, how quickly topics change, how some words convey emotion and other words merely suggest a thought. Before the stroke it never crossed my mind that something as simple as a breakfast conversation required the undivided attention of a fully functioning brain. But after the stroke it became a workout of astonishing proportions as my brain weighed a bevy of possibilities: That thought deserves a response, but not yet; that sentence signals the end of that person's contribution; now is the time to change the conversation, but maybe not; those words can be ignored; laughter might be a way to turn the page; when is it appropriate to ask for the butter? It is no wonder parents must teach manners over and over again to their children. Conversation, and the art of conversation, is no simple task. Kirby's advice about staying in controlled settings with just one or two people was not just well meaning, it was a neurologic necessity. I began to think of my brain as a two-cylinder engine trying to drive life's heavy-loaded Mercedes-- time and again it just didn't have the steam to keep up.

In the midst of all these events, of course, the "real world" continued to make its demands all of which had to be met by Connie. Fortunately I had disability insurance from the church and she had arranged for it to kick in after the stroke. At that time, none of us had any idea what a daunting struggle it would be to work with insurance companies that cannot possibly comprehend the stresses associated with serious injury. Although I had been through two heart attacks, and although Connie was the bookkeeper of our household, I had always perceived myself as the primary caregiver. The pain that makes it almost impossible for her to make it through a full day, did its best to eclipse the times we once climbed mountains and rowed the coast of Maine together. Now it all fell on her shoulders. Our income would be the Medicare disability payments she had been receiving since 1992, and my disability income. The church took up a generous collection to help tide us through as expenses increased and our capacity to meet them decreased.

The poet Richard Aldrich lived on the Maine coast and had been a colleague when Connie and I were teaching in Maine. Each day the waves hit, and then subsided, along the rocky shore beneath his home. He wrote a poem expressing that he heard them this way: "The ideal, the real, the ideal, the real," over and over again as each one reached for the shore, went as far as it could and then slipped back into the sea where it regrouped for yet another reach. Every day I would try to exceed expectations, only to hit reality's shore before slipping back into the land of rest. The more Connie saw the pattern the more she saw the need for "reality therapy" that neither she nor events could give. She called the Pioneer Medical Center and spoke with Barbara, an occupational therapist who had checked in on me when I was hospitalized for the seizure. Like most people, I had absolutely no idea what occupational therapy was. I associated it with tedious tasks, with learning to boil water or crocheting potholders. Just the words seemed like an assault. I had traveled to Lithuania once to report on a conference hosted by the Christian Children's Fund concerning the lives of people with disabilities in the Baltic nations. The stories of what happened to them during the communist era were heartbreaking. It was as though governments said, "Well, what are we going to do with you?" and then found a factory that would harness the least of their skills without taking into consideration what the person might want to do. When that failed, they just "forgot" about them, and many lived in their homes, completely unknown by their neighbors. I heard "occupational therapy" as consignment to a utilitarian life defined by the expectations and fears of others. It seemed to say, "We're going to do something with you." My impression, of course, had nothing to do with reality. In Barbara I found a listening ear, a voice of encouragement, and someone who asked what my life was like and wanted to trace where the lack of perception was taking me. With her I wasn't a problem. I was a person in transition. Often she was not promptly paid by the insurance company, which early on showed its aversion to things emotional and spiritual by simply not paying her.

She asked me to keep a daily journal and to share it with her when she came by the house on Wednesday afternoons. One day's entry still surprises me as my defiant reach for victory met an equally defiant reality.

Went over to church at ten o'clock to type an e-mail letter to the church. Did okay putting the letter together--but the connection kept going out--very frustrating. Left at 11:30 feeling exhausted--which means no spring to my thoughts. When I am at church all I can feel is what I'm not doing. Decided I would go to the Senior Center and did; almost nobody was there, but it was okay meeting people. They all say I look so good. I'm glad that the clunky brain has a good disguise.

Went to the Post Office--same thing; saw many people, greeted them and visa versa. That went okay. Loosing strength. Went to the Ben Franklin at 5:30 with Connie and saw its owners, and Diane--they are just two days from closing out. Big Timber will soon be a town of antiques and real estate offices, places for the rich but not for the people. We talked. Diane said I looked tired. I didn't step on words, but was close, and felt tense just relating the story; such a sense of guilt. When I tried to describe what had been lost Craig said with consummate kindness, "Now stop that, just rest." I found myself fighting back tears.

We went out to the car. I was so tired I was almost sick. The day--going to church, taking a phone call from a friend, the Senior Center, the Post Office, Craig and Diane--was too much--and some things I wanted to do I couldn't get done.

Once a week Barb listened patiently to my accounts of the day, sensing how frantically I was trying to deny the truth, patiently reminding me that rest was no shame. At the end of one day's journal she wrote:

> REMINDER TO LARRY
>
> *You see the big pictures, ask the big questions and know where you want to go. But remember, you have to master those baby steps first. You have to be able to do the basics SAFELY and consistently so you can get back to those issues.*
>
> *You need to relearn how to take care of yourself and keep yourself well. Then you can return to the work you love.*
>
> *Barb OT*

I thought, of course, that I had enough self-awareness to know how I was coming across to folks. But as Aesop so wisely informed us, we all carry two packs. We're aware of the one on the front, but the one on our backs can only be seen by others. One morning I "escaped" to Cole Drug where a group of friends always had coffee at exactly ten o'clock. I could hardly wait to see them again at the first booth sharing coffee and news of the day. I thought I spoke just fine, didn't miss many words, and made sense. Later Tom, a retired doctor, told me that after I left he had to wipe away tears. The missed words and confused sentence structure revealed damage I had yet to grasp.

Visits from friends continued, each of them wondering how he or she could be helpful to us. Gayle had been my piano teacher, and knew the rule barring me from trying to read music was one of the more exacerbating regulations. The piano had become as integral to my life as the banjo, and now it had been taken away. She was also an expert at Tai Chi and therapeutic massage. She thought, and I readily agreed, that adding Tai Chi to my morning exercises would be a good idea. It would help with my balance, and perhaps, just perhaps, its ancient rhythms would become a pathway to healing. She stopped by the house with massage pads in hand, showed me some basic Tai Chi motions, and offered a massage I was ever so glad to receive.

I had noticed that my balance wasn't as good as it might have been, but didn't think it was a real problem. Physical therapy certainly wasn't necessary--I could use my trusty Nordic Track, my various weights, and the Tai Chi moves she so kindly shared. But then, one day, I tried an exercise called "Holding Up the Sky." It involved slowly reaching up as high as I could with both arms, and then bending back my wrists as though I was actually holding up the sky. Then the trick was to shift my weight to my toes--something I found easier said than done. What surprised me, however, was the difference between my right arm and my left arm. My right arm stretched upward farther, and noticeably easier, than my left arm. My left shoulder felt thick whereas my right shoulder felt agile. I knew from the neurologist's tests that I had lost some feeling on my left side but hadn't realized it applied to the way muscles work as well. She gave me a massage on my left side, and its results were wonderful--temporary, but wonderful. Once again we were grateful for the ministry of a friend and the kindness of so many in our home town.

It should not be surprising that strange thoughts begin to emerge after a stroke. After all, many of the nerves that regulate "normal thinking" are no longer in place. Without their presence little thoughts become big ones, impulse masquerades as reason, and the daily string of collapses can't help but trigger depression. Studies have shown that half of all stroke patients find themselves in the slough of despond after their strokes. It even has a medical tag. "PSD" stands for Post Stroke Depression, and the literature is full of accounts revealing how common, how dangerous and how confusing it is for both the doctor and the patients.

"Most of the time," David said, "patients struggle with depression. But some will actually suffer from euphoria. I've had some patients who laugh uncontrollably practically all the time over absolutely nothing. That doesn't happen as much as depression though. It stems from changes in the brain and the dramatic changes in a person's life. There really are two realities that have dramatically changed. But I'm not really sure we should call it depression. I'd call it sadness. It is a sense of profound loss. Depression is when you have sad feelings but there is no reason for them. But the person who has had an injury or is in chronic pain has good reason to be sad."

"Perhaps it's better to see it as sorrow," I ventured.

"I think so. I'm not sure we need to give stroke or TBI patients to a psychiatrist. Now, of course, if disabling depression goes on for months and years that kind of care is warranted. But right after the injury, feeling a profound sense of loss is part of being a human being. That sadness may last for weeks, or months, or sometimes even years."

There is an entire genre of biblical literature devoted to sorrow. In our modern era we tend to deny sorrow its place preferring to say, "Move on" or "Move forward." In his exquisite book, *Road of the Tinkling Bell*, Tomihiro Hoshinou, a Japanese quadriplegic whose writings and paintings have inspired millions, writes about his preference for facing backwards when his wheelchair travels down the road. Instead of being pushed straight forward, he prefers to be pulled, allowing him to gaze into faces of those walking along the road. "It is said, 'Don't look back' or 'Live looking forward,'" he wrote. "I wonder if there is anyone who can live without looking back. Is it very admirable to go only looking forward? Of course we can't go forward if we always look back. If we feel guilty looking back, our daily life would be very stressful. It seems not all but some of our body structures are actually created for backward use." Sacred literature would make the same argument. Although a book devoted to only success might sell well, the Bible has an entire book named Lamentations and a first cousin named Ecclesiastes that emphasize that there is a time for joy, and a time for sorrow. The migration from sadness to hope is not a technique; it is not something that one simply "does." It is the work of life, and it takes time.

When I was in Moscow to report on the mission endeavors of the Russian Orthodox Church after the fall of communism, I happened to be at a monastery one day when a young women in a green dress came in and asked to speak with the priest. Not speaking Russian I had no idea what their conversation was about. When it was over, the two of them walked to the chapel and motioned for me to join them. Just the three of us were there. The bearded priest began a service that included prayers and liturgies in both song and the spoken word. The service was short, perhaps 20 minutes. When we left, I asked the priest what the service was about. The translator explained to me it was a memorial service. In their tradition there are four services following a death. First there is the funeral. Three weeks later, a second service is held. Three months later, a third service speaks a word of consolation to lingering grief. A year later, yet another service takes place. Grief takes time; lamentation needs its healing space. Post-stroke or TBI depression, stemming from a neurological rearrangement of life also needs time, healing space and medications to tame the newly unleashed power of despair.

Of the rules for the road to recovery one struck the core of my being. I had devoted my life to serving others through the written and spoken word. Take away the words and you take away life. Now they needed somebody else's permission lest they lead a person or a congregation astray. Kirby explained that the stroke had impaired the gift of judgment. Without it my words had the potential to inadvertently hurt somebody. In so many ways ministry is a matter of knowing what to say in situations that are often beyond words. A sermon goes through thousands of filters—what is the text saying? What might the congregation hear? What mis-impressions must be challenged? What do we need to hear? It all calls for discernment and careful judgment.

Like Pandora who had been instructed to not open the box, and did so anyway, I found the temptation to send e-mails overwhelming. Connie, of course, found out and lovingly asked me why I had repeated myself so many times in the course of a single e-mail.

"I did?"

"Yes."

"I didn't know that."

"But you did."

"I did?"

"Yes, and you just repeated yourself again."

Like it or not there was a compelling reason for the rule.

Christmas was just around the corner. The kindness of the congregation, and the leadership they evidenced Sunday after Sunday as they shared the word, and the power of the season itself, all spoke of life. Kirby and Julie could not have been kinder. Knowing that not being at church on Christmas Eve would be heartbreaking, they invited us to spend Christmas Eve with them and their baby, Luke. We drove over to their house, had a wonderful supper, and good conversation. As the Hebrews so poignantly observed, hospitality is a form of worship. And so, in the bleak midwinter we celebrated Christmas.

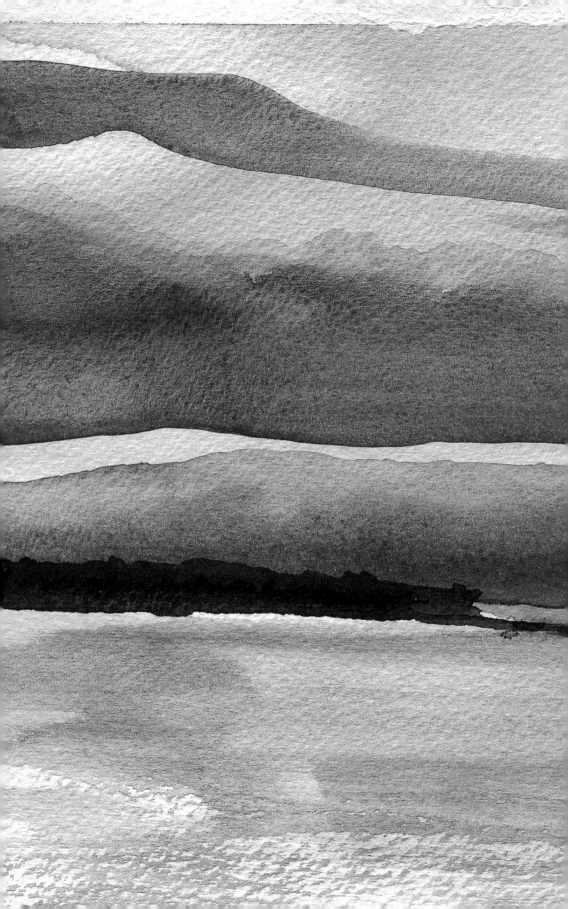

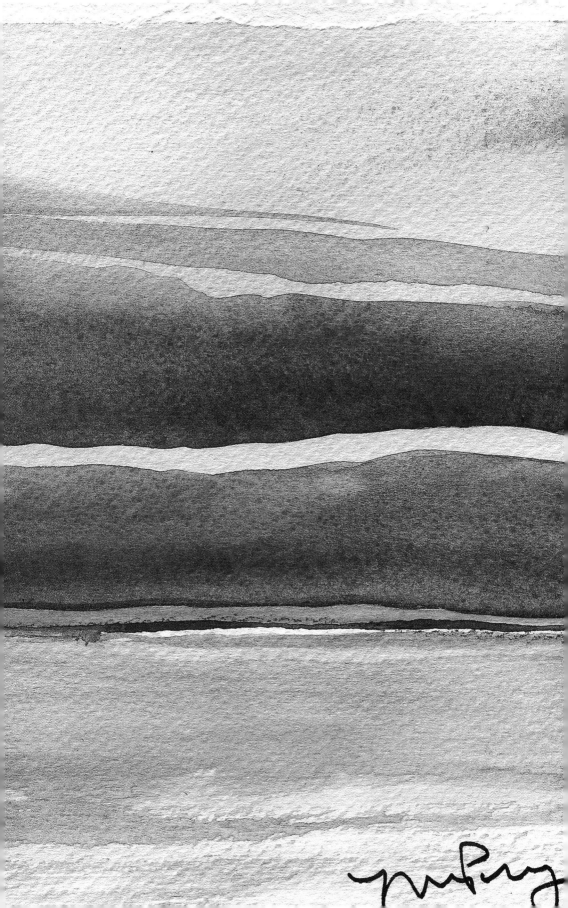

chapter nine
what's left

•••

It seemed as though we were out of options. Neither hospitalization had turned the clock back. We didn't belong in the house of New Hope. The extent of Antarctica's reach kept revealing itself in an absence of feeling, the loss of music, confused clocks and fatigue that claimed the day. There were, however, questions that needed to be answered. How much cognitive ability had been lost? In January, 2004, two months after my stroke, Kirby spoke with St. Vincent's Behavioral Health Center whose psychologists had been specifically trained to make such an evaluation. The receptionist said it would be at least a three-hour exam, and warned us that it would be exhausting. Nevertheless, we were both anxious to determine how much of "me" was left. We had a sense that the more complete our understanding the clearer our pathway would be. The exam would answer the two questions that framed the historic mission and ministry of the United Church of Christ and its predecessors: In light of these circumstances, What good can be done? And by what means?

We drove to Billings and arrived at the center, which was housed in an innocuous building not far from the hospital. Connie checked us in, showing the small cards with an insurance company's name and number that spell the difference between life and death for so many Americans. Having passed inspection, we took a seat. I immediately began to wonder if we were in the right place. There were three or four people sitting in the waiting room, most reading tired magazines with their eyes facing down to avoid a glance of recognition. It was not a place for conversation. The name of the office seemed odd to me. What is a Behavioral Health Center? Had I misbehaved? Were the other people waiting in the room also stroke survivors? Or was it a counseling facility that treated mental illness? Part of me wanted to say, "I'm not here because I'm depressed. I had a stroke. You too?" I am ashamed of that reaction as I look back on it. Depression is not something to be ashamed of, and mental illness is as intrinsic a disease as diabetes or cancer. But take away a billion or so cells that balance the raw run of emotion and the sharp edge of prejudice abruptly presents itself with startling power.

"Mr. and Mrs. Pray?"

"Come this way please."

A middle-aged woman with a warm smile welcomed us into her office. She was a trained psychologist who also worked with stroke patients to assess how severe their damage had been. She was licensed to give the tests that would determine cognitive ability. We had never met her before. There were two comfortable chairs in front of her desk. For some reason it struck me that there were no distractions on her desk – no pile of papers, no mementos, nothing to distinguish it from any other business-like desk. She invited us to sit down and then did so herself behind the desk. Connie sat down but I remained in an awkward stand. She again invited me to sit down, but I still remained standing. Connie looked at me, and asked me directly to sit down. At her request I finally took my seat. Why had I resisted? I had been shot down by the stroke, by the neurologist, by the seizure, and by New Hope. Perhaps I was simply resisting any possibility of being shot down again. Or perhaps I just didn't know how to "fit in." But David had a different take on the awkward moment.

"The bulk of the brain's right hemisphere, where your stroke occurred, processes spatial information," he said. "I'm wondering if the damage it suffered didn't make it difficult for you to initiate action. People with brain injuries often know what they're supposed to do but they can't initiate the action necessary to do it. You knew you were supposed to sit down, but couldn't start the action. When Connie helped you and said, 'Sit down,' that started the motor sequence which allowed you to comply. To me that explains your standing. It isn't that you were rude, you just couldn't initiate the appropriate action. Did you have initiation problems in other areas?"

"Yes," I answered. "It was strange that although I knew I should be having meetings with the church leadership, I just couldn't, or didn't, call a meeting to map out the months ahead of us. I kept thinking I needed to meet with them but didn't."

"Well, that's it," said David. "People with right brain strokes can often talk about what they need to do, but they can't follow through. You knew you should call a meeting, and didn't. Or you knew you should have sat down, but until Connie reached out to actually start the motor sequence, you couldn't."

I later started using the word "traction" to describe the situation. Each day began with plans, but the plans just couldn't gain traction. Sometimes I would sit down at the computer to write and find myself just staring at it waiting for something to happen. Entire days would pass without traction. Routine took the place of creative endeavor. Sloth is one of the seven deadly sins, and my ordination vows were clear: aimlessness and idleness are not trifling matters. Indeed the Statement of Faith of the United Church of Christ notes that "God seeks in holy love to save His creation from evil, aimlessness and sin." Ministry is an open-ended calling that always presents another thing to do, another book to read, another call to make. "Slow down," I had always been told. "Good idea", I'd say, "just as soon as I've finished this…and that…and that." Finally life forced my hand, requiring me to do what I'd been asked to do so many times.

It was time for the interview to find traction.

"I understand you have had a stroke," the doctor said after I'd finally taken my seat. I nodded my head. "I'm really sorry that happened." Her tone and words could not have been kinder.

"The purpose of today is to see which parts of your brain have been injured and what we might be able to do to remedy the situation. I can tell you for sure that with work things will get better. I've seen so many patients make so much progress. So though I know things seem grim right now, they will get better.

"Can you tell me just a bit about what happened?"

In the flat and emotionless voice, I recounted the early days of the stroke. I told her about the tree that suddenly lost its leaves. From time to time I missed words, apologizing each time I mispronounced something simple –saying

"Povember" instead of November or "schpittle" for hospital. Before a word emerged incorrectly I tried to "step" on it, giving me a chance to make a correction. Sometimes I could head the mispronunciations off at the pass; sometimes I couldn't. Sometimes outward back came words, and sometimes they came out right. From time to time Connie filled in part of the story.

"One day at the hospital he just walked out," she said. The psychologist nodded her head. She had evidently heard of that before.

"You've been a pastor?"

"Yes."

"In Big Timber?"

"Yes."

"What denomination?"

"Congregational," I said. "Congregationalists are part of the United Church of Christ."

"How are you feeling most of the time," she asked.

"I feel fine, but it's not me. It's as though I'm somebody else. Words don't give themselves anymore. And my voice is wrong. It's not my voice. And I tire so easily."

"That's perfectly normal," she said.

"Have you been depressed?"

"Yes," I said, listening again to the voice that wasn't mine. "I'd say I've been depressed. Everybody said it was a miracle that I'd survived but I do keep wondering why the stroke didn't take all of me. Mostly I'm tired and don't really recognize myself. It's like I died."

"Do you think he's been depressed?" she asked Connie.

"Yes," she said. "He really is."

"That's a good thing," she said.

"It is?"

"Yes. It means your brain is beginning to grasp what happened. If you weren't depressed it would mean you were living without much awareness. Strokes always take away a sense of self-awareness. So I know it sounds strange, but depression after a stroke is actually a good sign. It means your brain is beginning to recognize what happened. You got hit really hard, and now your brain is beginning to sense a huge loss. Depression is one manifestation of that recognition. A deep sense of loss is appropriate."

So Behavioral Health was the right building. I should have said to those waiting in the lobby, "I'm here for depression, are you?" Never in my life would I have thought that depression is a good thing.

And then she asked the key question.

"What would your goals for recovery be?"

"I want my life back," I said. Each word carried volumes of power. There were no syllables to trip me up. Five words told the story, each wrapped in purpose and anger. There were no meanings to mistake, no hidden implications to uncover, no mispronunciations to revamp. The message was pure emotion and pure will.

"I want my life back."

"I do not want a new life.

"I love the life I had.

"I love the church I've been called to serve.

"I love Big Timber, Montana.

"I want my life back."

The words were clear but even as I spoke them I knew they also betrayed the truth. For a Christian there is no such thing as "my life." Whatever we accomplish, whoever we become, however we serve reflects the intersection of the Spirit with the concrete personality of self. To God be the glory, we sing Sunday after Sunday. "You are the potter, we are the clay," we sing echoing the lines of Jeremiah. We enter worship to be relieved of the burden of self, to discern the palpable presence of God in shaping our lives. Quietly, reverently, we sing:

> Spirit of the living God, fall afresh on me;
> Melt me, mold me, fill me, use me
> Spirit of the living God, fall afresh on me.

For 13 years Connie and I wrote and produced the *Calendar of Prayer* for the United Church of Christ. It involved reading thousands of mission statements, corresponding with missionaries around the world in days before e-mail made such correspondence ever-so easy. Each day we wrote about a church, or a mission agency somewhere in the world or at home. The postman often wondered just what it was we did, when he delivered strange-looking bags of tea from a Tibetan refugee center, and letters from Lesotho, East Timor, and Mozambique. The stories were always a source of inspiration. One mission statement struck us with its exceptional clarity: "God accepts us just the way we are, and loves us too much to leave us there." Life is never owned by a person. It is always open to the Spirit's leading. Even when all is well, God may have another step in mind.

To have said, "I want my life back" was a sharp and selfish denial of that truth. My five word sentence reverberated with stunning clarity and spiritual treason. Some day I would need to surrender. But now was not the time.

Our get acquainted interview was over, and it was time for the test to begin. I could feel Connie's apprehension, and worried I had made the counselor uncomfortable with my anger-laced words. I didn't mean to do that.

"Let's start the test," she said.

She took out a series of cards, each of which had a three dimensional drawing. In each triangle, rectangle or circle something was missing. On some cards the missing piece was obvious as when a triangle didn't have a bottom or a circle lacked part of its arc. Beside each drawing there were three or four lines, one of which would fix the drawing. The test was seemingly simple. Would line A, B, or C be the correct answer? I knew it was going to be a challenge. Mechanical matters, to say nothing of following directions, had always been difficult for me. I had no idea how my high school friends took motors apart and then put them back together. They had no idea why I cared so deeply about the cadence of a sentence and loved nothing more than reading Shakespeare. But this was not a time to quote Chaucer. It was time to take a test.

The first set of cards was easy. But soon the drawings became complex and I had to begin guessing.

"She was testing your matrix reasoning," said David. "She used the Wechsler Adult Intelligence Scale. It has both a verbal and a performance component. With a right-brained stroke we would expect a person to do far better on the verbal part than the performance part. Anything spatial would have been a challenge for you given what happened to your parietal lobe. That test asked you to locate things in space, to see how things fit together, and to visualize what happens if you rotate a pattern. If you had correctly answered most of them it would have shown that you didn't have too much damage to the parietal lobe. The more you missed, the greater the damage."

I had no idea how I'd scored on the spatial test. Although she had made it clear the test wasn't a competition, I wanted to be successful. I wanted to win. I wanted my life back. My strength began to ebb.

"How are you doing?" she asked.

"Fine," I answered.

"Ready for the next?"

"Okay."

"This time I am going to show you a series of faces, and then I will go through them a second time and ask you which ones you have seen."

"Okay."

Each four-by-six card had a full-color face on it. She gave me about five seconds to study each card. I couldn't help but wonder, "Who are these people? What are their lives like? How did they ever get their picture taken? What might their names be? How old are they? What country do they live in? Did their parents say it was okay to have their picture taken?" One was a Chinese girl, maybe 15 years old. Another picture must have been taken in Scotland or Ireland as the girl had red hair, freckles and pale white skin. Another was an East African, or Mexican, looking lonely, even a little bit scared. What happened to her? Was she okay? Yet another might have had Down Syndrome. Yet another had his head tilted just a bit to the side. Was he Egyptian? Or was he from southern India?

I tried to concoct a story for each face, but I no sooner invented a story than she turned to another card which had a different face requiring a different story. Soon she had been through the entire deck.

"Now, I'll show you a set of pictures, and you tell me which faces you remember."

"Okay."

The first card came up. I didn't remember it. Then the next. Had I seen her before? Then the next. She had to be the girl from Ireland. I had seen her before. Maybe.

"Yes."

"Okay." "This one?"

"I think, but I'm not sure."

"How about this one?"

"No."

I knew I was striking out. My mind was a complete blank, no matter how hard I tried to remember a story, a look, the tilt of a head, or complexion of a child I kept coming up empty. More strength drained away.

"That sequence tested your nonverbal memory," said David. "And it isn't easy. She showed you 28 faces at two seconds a face. Then she showed a different set with those 28 faces mixed in, and then she asked if you recognized the face from the first deck. And then, after 30 minutes, she showed another set of faces some of which you would have seen before, and others that were new. You had to identify the ones you recognized. That tested your delayed recall. Here again, the damage to your right brain would have made this a real challenge."

I was glad when she gathered the cards together and put them back into a drawer or perhaps her briefcase.

"Okay," she said. "Let's go to the next test."

"Okay," I said.

She took out another set of cards that had a series of scenes drawn on them. The pictures reminded me of elementary school textbooks which showed Dick, Jane and their trusty dog Spot. She wanted to know if I could interpret the scene. These were easy. Yes, the family was sharing a barbecue. Yes, two kids were playing on a swing. Yes there were clouds in the sky. It all made sense. It was not hard to draw inferences from the pictures. These cards felt like a kind of reprieve.

Then it was time for the next test.

"I'm going to say 15 word sequences very slowly," she said. You can repeat after me if you'd like."

"Okay."

"What we want to see is how many sequences you can remember."

"Okay."

"Here goes:

HOUSE CLOUD

ELEPHANT BRICK

RACCOON PAPER

DOOR RAG

SPICE CAR

The words had absolutely nothing to do with each other. I listened carefully; repeated after her; and tried to invent some kind of link that would remind me of a sequence. Raccoons do get into papers in the trash, so that one was easy. Elephants probably wouldn't like bricks, I said to myself. But just as soon as I tried to weave them together, she'd say the next two words. She repeated the list four times. And then she said only the first word and waited to see if I could remember the second.

"Elephant," she said.

"Brick," I said.

"Spice," she said. "Rag," I said.

"That test is specifically designed to not give you cues," said David. "The words aren't meaningful and that's the whole point. They weren't like LION GROWL, or WIND TORNADO. The context couldn't give you a clue. It tested the left temporal lobe of your brain which is responsible for language. We would have expected you do to better with these verbal tests. But they would still be a challenge, and the stroke still affected how you did. You wouldn't do as well even with verbal things as you would have before the stroke. A stroke like yours impacts your entire system even though the specific damage is to the right side of your brain."

There was yet another test.

"Ready?" she asked gently. She could sense my fatigue.

"Whew," I said.

I want my life back. If this is what it would take to get my life back I would do it so help me Hannah.

"Okay, let's go," I said.

"I'm going to read you a paragraph two times. After I've done that I'd like you to retell me the story with all its details."

"Okay." She picked out a card and began to read:

Ralph Thompson of Tacoma was watching television and wanted to go out. A weather report on the news said a storm would be moving into the area in four or five hours with four inches of rain, and it could bring hail. Ralph knew the rain would be a major problem in the city and beyond, so he decided to cancel his plans. He called Sue and asked if she would like to go to the movies with him before the rain started to fall. Sue thanked him for the invitation but she already had plans. So Ralph changed his plans again and walked to the video store where he rented three videos and settled in for the weekend.

The story seemed simple enough. She read it again. This time I tried to imprint each detail in my mind: Tacoma; five o'clock; three inches of rain, not one, not two but three read'em three inches of rain; Sue, her name was Sue, traffic problems, traffic, traffic, traffic problems; Hail; Plans." She asked me to retell the story.

"Joe came home from his job in San Francisco and turned on the television which forecasted a lot of rain. So did the six o'clock weather report. He called Mary and she said that much rain would a problem be. She didn't want to go out with him. So he got some videos for the weekend."

This time she told me what I'd left out and what I added. "Three inches of rain, traffic problems, change of plans, Mary had plans, three videos." Hmmm....I got the gist of the story but not its life. Then it was time for two more stories. Each time I got most of the story, but left out the details that gave it lift and life. By now I was completely exhausted, as was Connie who patiently stayed for the entire exam.

"That test had lots of verbal contexts," said David. "And context is a different kind of learning, a different kind of recognition. Without context understanding is hit or miss, so the ability to interpret events in their context is important. Having you retell those stories was one way to measure how much of that capacity you had lost."

It was time to wrap up the afternoon.

As David and I pieced together the test experience I suddenly wondered if this post-stroke test was an IQ test. For some reason, I assumed it was different. A person receives an IQ test once in his or her life. IQ tests had always raised a red flag in my mind. What does a 120 mean? What does a 90 mean? Does it hold any spiritual significance? Isn't it an inherently elitist test, giving power to some and taking power away from others? If life is a matter of loving God and neighbor, what possible impact could an IQ test have on the fundamental commandments?

"Was that an IQ test?" I asked David. I was sure he would say, "No." I wanted him to say, "No, it is a post-stroke test that is quite different from the IQ test you took when you were a child."

Instead he said, "The test you received was the Wechsler Adult Intelligence Scale II, and it is an IQ test. In fact it is the granddaddy of all IQ tests. I would guess that you performed in the low 90s which would have been a significant drop for you. You should have been in the 125 range before the stroke. The drop from 125 to 90 is huge. No wonder you could scarcely recognize yourself. The person you were in thought and perception before the stroke no longer existed. So much was taken away that you really did become a different person."

It had indeed been a long afternoon and we had a long drive home. The psychologist had said it would take several weeks to compile the results.

"I just want to remind you," she said, as we prepared to leave, "that progress is possible. Things are going to get better for you. Therapy can make a real difference, so you're not 'stuck' if you don't want to be."

"But where do we get that therapy?" Connie asked. "We went to New Hope and they said he was too well to be part of that program."

"And the neurologist said the brain cells that are gone are gone forever," I said.

"Yes, but with therapy other cells can take over their functions."

"I just want my life back. That's all."

"I know," she said.

"What about Headway?" Connie asked. Kirby had told us about Headway, a cognitive therapy program at St. Vincent Healthcare. We did not realize then that

Headway was one of only two such programs in Montana, and that no such program existed in Idaho, Wyoming, or the Dakotas. It struck us that once again God had brought us to the right place. When we came to Montana we found a pain specialist in Billings who agreed to work with Connie. He had a level of compassion, understanding and medical insight that ironically we had not been able to find in Minnesota, a state filled with medical expertise. It was almost as though the call to Big Timber was destined to renew my call to ministry but also to give Connie the medical care she increasingly needed. And now we miraculously found ourselves just 80 miles away from one of the few programs in the country that specializes in cognitive therapy. For years I had been saying to Sunday School kids who were about to disappear into their teenage years, "In your life there will be times you fall away from God. But God will never fall away from you." I had fallen away from the capacity to pray, but perhaps what I'd preached to the kids was true, God had not fallen away from us. There was a place called Headway and it was only 80 miles away.

"How do we get into Headway?" Connie asked.

"I'll send the results of this exam over to them with a recommendation for you. Then they will give you a complete evaluation and determine whether or not you're a candidate for the program."

We both said, "Okay."

"Thank you," we said and left the office. Connie got into the driver's seat because I was not allowed to drive for fear of another seizure. And then unbridled emotion began to spill out.

"I don't trust that," I said. I have no idea where the venom came from but anger seeped through my voice.

"Why?"

"I don't know. I just don't." There was an edge to my voice. I had always considered myself a fairly gentle soul. Like Rex Harrison in *My Fair Lady*, "I had the milk of human kindness by the quart in every vein." But sweet milk turns sour when taken out of its element. Could Headway make sour milk sweet? We didn't know. The psychologist's kind words about healing should have been reassuring, but I somehow could not trust her.

Connie made arrangements for a meeting with Headway, and we waited for a written evaluation of my testing. It didn't arrive and didn't arrive. I finally called and asked for it.

"It's very complicated," said the psychologist who administered the test. "I don't think you would be able to understand the numbers and all of the concepts. It basically shows the damage that comes from a right-brain stroke. Your functional level is far down from what I believe it once was, so yes a lot has been lost, but not everything." I still wanted to see it in writing and asked her to send it to us anyway. She finally, and reluctantly for some reason, agreed to send it and, sure enough, the numbers and graphs were indecipherable.

The morning paper took on a new significance. Every crossword became an exercise in restoration. I had heard that working crossword puzzles had the power to hold dementia and Alzheimer's disease at bay. Then I'd try a Sudoku puzzle. On Mondays they were easy, and some of the time I could get them. When I failed I redrew the puzzle on a clean sheet of paper and then used multi-colored pens to aid in the search and to try to find a solution. "Practice makes perfect," I'd say. Everything I did turned into a bit of therapy, a way to explore what had happened and a way to set things right.

Before the stroke I had been invited to address a group of healers trained and gathered by the Interfaith Health Program in Atlanta. The IHP crowd understood that the church must have something to do with healing. Each of the people I had interviewed for the book on Boundary Leadership, had done just that. I could hardly wait to share the gist of the many interviews I had conducted with boundary leaders in Norway, South Africa, Germany and throughout the United States. Each one had became a friend, even though we had never met except over the telephone. Each one had such a compelling insight to share, and profound experience in navigating the boundary between "what is" and "what could be." To share their stories in person, as well as in the book that would later emerge, and to be once again amidst a community of healers, would be a cause for celebration.

The trip, however, was out of the question. Kirby was concerned that if I tried it I might very well never come home. It would be an uncontrolled setting, I would have to interpret the million and one regulations of air travel and would need days, or weeks, to recover from the raw expenditure of energy. It was a no go. On the tractionless day I was to have been in Atlanta, the phone rang. It was Gary, calling from the meeting saying that everyone wished me well and had held us in prayer. I didn't know that Connie and one of the kids had called him, both to give a report and to ask if he'd make a call.

One never knows just what it is that unleashes tears. Since the stroke I had not wept. I had been angry; I had been sad; I had been thankful for the kindness of so many people at church; but I had not wept. After the call, I put down the phone and began to sob. My heart was with those people, just as my heart was with the people of the First Congregational Church in Big Timber, Montana. The wider world had always inspired local ministry, just as local ministry guided and inspired the wider world. There had always been a way to do both. But reality told me something different. "No," it said on both levels. "They're there, and you're here. And we don't know if there is a way to be with either the church or IHP again. Only time will tell." Connie heard my sobs, came over, and we embraced, both of us aware that finally the depth of this strange new world had hit home.

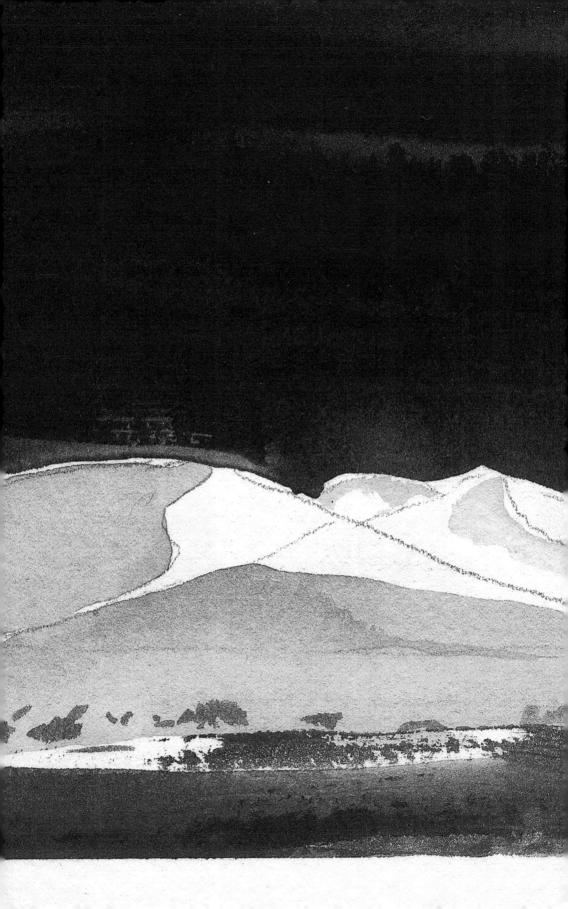

chapter ten
recognition and reassembly

• • •

Connie called Headway to make an appointment. A woman named Mandi fielded her call and together they set a date. "You should plan on staying for several hours," she told Connie. "We want to acquaint you with the program, and also make an evaluation that will provide a base line." We could scarcely imagine there could be yet more tests to take, and wondered if we would have the strength to go through yet another day in Billings. Connie then learned that the case manager had just left Headway.

"Does that mean the program is falling apart?" she asked, drawing on her years of working with foundations and corporations in New York City. When the principal leaves, it's not always a good sign, to say the least. Connie wanted to know if he had resigned, if something had gone awry, or if his departure was nothing more than an orderly transition.

"No, we've got it all covered," Mandi said. "All the staff is here and the program is in good shape. We look forward to seeing you. We're on the lower level of the Yellowstone Medical Arts Building West. It's right across the street from the Emergency Room."

We shelved our concerns and when the day finally arrived we headed for the Magic City, as Billings is sometimes called. An attendant offered to park our car and we agreed. We walked inside, found an elevator, waited for its door to open, went inside and pressed the button marked LL. Sometimes the most important decisions in life require the fewest words. Wedding vows take but a moment to say but have the power to shape the rest of one's life. We did not speak as the elevator began its descent, but we both knew the button we had just pressed was taking us, for better or for worse, into another world. Perhaps we would find healing. Perhaps not. We had no choice but to find out.

When the doors opened we faced a stunning painting in a small hallway. The landscape portrayed blue mountains, fields with purple edges and the intense red and orange sky that often graces winter. It immediately reminded me of my years of coaching cross country in Maine. At the end of the season, when the weather grew cold, the hills we ran across held those same shades. It was a real painting. Thankfully, the hospital didn't use motel art. We gazed at the painting and followed a short hallway to the Rehabilitative Services lobby. Interestingly enough, there was no sign for Headway. Most of the people in the lobby had one kind of brace or another. Some had walkers, a few had wheelchairs. For a second I wondered what a brain brace might look like. We checked in with the secretary behind the counter who assured us we were in the right place and asked us to take a seat.

Connie had brought everything we had received by mail from Headway about the program, including a basic brochure describing its services. The brochure said that the average stay was three or four months. It seemed inconceivably long. It had already been almost two months since my stroke, and the neurologist said I needed to take three months off. February would be time to go back to work. I had three or four weeks to heal. Whatever they said, I would do it.

A door opened and a Korean woman asked, "Are the Prays here?"

"Are you Mandi?" Connie asked.

"Yes, glad to see you. Come this way."

She led us into a hallway that then went three separate ways. To the right we saw a small swimming pool. To the left there was a small indoor track and gym with all kinds of weight equipment. Mandi led us down the corridor directly in front of us, past rooms full of ACE bandages, examination tables, and charts showing skeletal structure. She then led us down another long hallway with beautiful Native American prints along its walls. Once again I was impressed with the art. Good things happen in places with good art. It had always struck me that the walls of elementary school classrooms are generally alive with color, with finger paintings or cutouts made by the kids themselves. By the time kids reach junior high school art has been replaced by posters, and in high school all sense of design and creativity has frequently gone by the wayside. I found the art reassuring. Headway was a creative place.

At the end of the hallway there was a double door. Mandi opened it and we stepped into a large carpeted rectangular room.

"This is our day room," she said. A light beech, or maybe birch, table, that could easily seat eight people stood in the center of the room. Not far from it there were two or three other tables, several file cabinets, and a make-shift office cubicle. One wall had an eraser board with the first names of patients and their daily schedule. The board immediately reminded me of patient boards in intensive care facilities. After both my heart attacks I had seen my name written upon such a board. To have one's name eventually crossed off was a sign of either healing or the profound absence of healing. Either way, such boards denoted serious business.

Facing the board there was a couch, two softly padded recliners and a small coffee table. Other than the schedule board there was nothing to indicate it as a treatment room. It was an altogether comfortable and social environment. I did not realize at the time that it was carefully designed to be just that way. Other hospitals sometimes relegate cognitive patients to nearly antiseptic rooms whose white walls and linoleum floors serve to separate one from the ebb and flow of everyday life. Headway made no attempt to follow the medical model.

Mandi indicated we should take a seat and then introduced us to the staff who sat around the table anticipating the intake conference. For the first time we met David Gumm; Chris, the speech therapist; Nicole, the occupational therapist; and Carol, the physical therapist. They had received the report of my IQ evaluation and had discussed it before our arrival.

Mandi spoke a bit about cognitive rehabilitation, emphasizing that she had seen many people both recover and shape new lives. Some of the Headway patients suffered traumatic brain injury from an external source such as a fall or an automobile accident, and others suffered injury from a stroke. All the Headway patients were outpatients.

We had but one question: Could they help us? It was an "us" question. The person I once knew had died; the person Connie knew had changed. Neither of us knew how to adjust.

Can you help us?

Yes, they said, they thought they could. Therapy would be frustrating, difficult, and painfully slow to measure. But they knew what they were doing. Speaking to Connie, David emphasized that the family plays a key role in recovery from brain injury. He welcomed her as an active participant. They also explained that all patients are assigned a social worker. We wondered if that might involve an extra charge, but no, they assured us it was an integral part of the program. Rehabilitation had a physical, an emotional, a mental and vocational sphere. Curiously enough there was no chaplain.

When could we start? If the insurance company approved, we could start in a week or two. I assumed it would be a five-days-a-week endeavor. Eight hours a day would be fine. Twelve would even be better. But such heroic thoughts were born of denial not reality. I could scarcely read the paper before a day would slip away into oblivion, to say nothing of carrying on a conversation in groups. I was not the first patient to say, "Couldn't we do this faster?" or the first to deny the full implications of a stroke or TBI. In reassuring tones the Headway team said that given my case, three hours a day, three days a week, Monday, Tuesday and Thursday, would be best. Wednesdays and weekends would provide time for recovery. It never occurred to me that "given my case" reflected their understanding of the full scope of the damage.

"Are you sure that's enough?" I asked, still eager to up the ante.

"Yes," they said. "It's more than you think."

Therapy would begin at 11:00, break for lunch, and then start up again at 1:00. Transportation would be a problem as I still couldn't drive, and Connie's disability made that many trips almost an impossibility. But there were always people needing to go to Billings, and many in the church offered to lend a hand. We could not have been more blessed by friends and congregation. The conversation lulled.

"Let me show you the whole facility," said Mandi. She took us into the gym, explained that most of my therapy would take place in the day room, showed us where the restrooms were, and opened a cabinet file in which each patient had a colored folder filled with exercise sheets and papers. She then showed us a small kitchen and explained I'd be spending time in it as part of occupational therapy. I couldn't help but flash back to junior high school where the girls went to home economics and the boys went to shop. How strange to suddenly have a "home ec" room. We went back to the day room and Mandi said it was time for the staff to do some evaluations. The CAT scan: an evaluation; the MRI: an evaluation; the IQ test: an evaluation; the drawing of a clock: an evaluation; how many more could there be? There were four. The first would be with Chris, the speech therapist.

"Ready?" she asked.

"Let's go." She led me down the art-filled hallway and asked me to sit down in a small office. I knew nothing about speech therapy save the story of Helen Keller and Annie Sullivan. Between them life found a language. Perhaps my language could also find life. First, however, she needed to make her own assessment. She heard the drone and the mispronunciations that intruded from time to time, but made no comment about either one.

"I'm going to give you a minute or so, and I'd like you to say all the words you can that begin with the letter 'S'" she said.

"Okay," I said. It seemed like a no-brainer. I'd been a writer and a speaker most of my life. Certainly coming up with 50 words that began with the letter "S" would be no problem. Thousands of words begin with "S." What could be simpler? All I had to do was start and the words would flow like a river.

"Okay," she said. "Go."

I nodded my head and tried to think of a word that began with the letter "S". To my utter astonishment, no such word appeared. Not a single one. Nothing happened. I looked at her. I tried again to find a word. Nothing happened. My brain was like the little wheel on an Apple Computer that says "I'm processing, I'm searching, I'm processing, I'm looking, but haven't found anything yet." When something is wrong with the computer the wheel can rotate for hours. Finally, after perhaps ten seconds, I finally said "SAND."

I tried to find a second. Another ten seconds passed. Finally, almost in panic,

I thought of "SALAD." An eternity passed before I could find a third. Chris sensed my astonishment. I could talk but couldn't find a single word.

"That's hard, isn't it," she said.

"I can't believe it."

"Let me tell you what's happened," she said. "Your brain is like a giant filing cabinet. Before your stroke all of its information had a folder, a drawer, a place, and your brain knew exactly where to find things. But the stroke took all of those files and threw them helter-skelter across the room. The papers are all over the place. There isn't any order anymore. So when you search for a specific word your brain has no idea where to go. It might be here; it might be there; it might be anywhere. That's why it is taking you so long to find a word.

"But then why can I talk?"

"That's different," she said. "The brain is so complex it works in many, many ways so a string of words, or a sentence, is different from searching for a single word. But I'll bet you often find yourself stumbling on words or using the wrong one. Is that right?"

"Yes." I was both impressed with the extent of her knowledge and still dumbfounded that I could not find even six words beginning with "S".

"It's just unbelievable," I said. I knew life had changed but had no idea my brain, the giver of words, had lost its capacity to search and find. Clearly therapy would be a matter of picking up all the spilled files, going through them one by one, designing a new filing system, and becoming reacquainted with the gift, the precious gift, of language. The monotone would have to wait.

We went back into the day room, and Chris handed me over to Carol who led me to the gym. She asked me to walk a straight line, and watched me carefully to see if I could maintain balance. Then she asked me to copy her as she walked the line sideways, moving one foot across the other. The motion was left over right, then right swinging behind the left foot until it came up along side it, and then left behind right, then right over left, and so on. It reminded me of square dance classes when I was in junior high school. Once you got the hang of an allemande left and a do-si-do dances were a snap. But every time I tried to copy Carol's steps I'd get lost. No matter how hard I tried to "get it right" I couldn't coordinate my motions.

"Good," she'd say if I got a few steps right.

"Okay," I'd say, "I think I've got it." But then my feet would get bollixed up yet again. I'd thought my balance and coordination were pretty good. But Carol's test, like Chris', showed unmistakably that my self awareness wasn't exactly sharp. In fact, it was way off base.

"The miracle is that you were able to move at all," said David. "Most people with strokes have hemisplegia. If it is a right brain stroke they can't move the left side of their body. If it is a left brain stroke they can't move, or sometimes even feel, the right side of their body. Why you didn't have hemisplegia nobody knows. The truth is you shouldn't be walking. You have dodged so many bullets it is incredible. Have you seen the movie *Mr. and Mrs. Smith*? There is all of this shooting, and nobody gets hit. You're like that. Or you're like the chief in *Little Big Man* who goes right into battle believing he is invisible and so he never gets hit. That's you.

"The reason you felt that thickness in your left shoulder, and the reason you were having problems with your balance is that a lot of the wires that coordinate motion, or give you spatial awareness, were missing. The miracle is that you could move at all given the extent of your stroke." Although David had read the reports from Kirby and the various neurologists, he had not seen the actual MRI. I brought it in one day to show him. We went into a conference room that had a back-lit screen and clipped in the film. "My God," he said, almost losing his balance at the extent of Antarctica's reach. The damage was overwhelming, the fact that I had survived at all was nothing short of a miracle.

Carol led me back into the day room. It was time for an occupational therapy test. The words still had a Stalinist tinge despite my work with Barbara. I had once traveled to Lithuania for a conference on the status of people with disabilities in the Baltic Nations after the fall of communism. Not knowing what to do with "them" the state gave "them" something, anything, to do. They were kept out of sight. The stories were heartbreaking. Occupational therapy seemed like a threat instead of a way to enhance the skills, hopes and even dreams of stroke or TBI survivors. At its core it is a spiritual discipline looking for ways to harness whatever capacities are left after a traumatic injury or neglected in the course of everyday life. Nicole wasn't a "Home Ec" teacher.

"Okay," she said as we entered the small kitchen, "what we're going to do is make macaroni and cheese and see how that goes." Surely I could cook Kraft macaroni and cheese. I love to cook, to bake bread, to try new recipes. Our kids were almost shy about bringing friends over for dinner because their Dad never cooked "regular food." If there was a recipe for Moroccan lamb, Iraqi tabouli, Lithuania's version of bagels, or marinated tongue, I'd cook it. They were thankful beyond measure for the many times their mother rescued them from their father's exotic Iranian stew with a down home meatloaf or a pizza. Boiling water for macaroni and cheese would be "duck soup."

Nicole sat down at the small formica table and watched me go about the appointed task. The cabinets were all carefully labeled: SPICES, DISHES, UTENSILS, MEASURING CUPS, POTS AND PANS, and so on. I knew, without even reading the directions, that water had to be boiled. I checked the directions to impress Nicole, measured out two cups of water, poured them into a pan and turned on the burner.

What's next.

Oh yes, the butter. I put everything out as though I was a *mise en place* chef.

"I love to cook," I said.

"Do you?" she said, watching every move and noting it on her chart. I later learned that Nicole's notes were the most meticulous of all the therapists. She didn't miss anything. Neither she, nor the program, could afford to. The physics and chemistry of cooking involve risk and must be carefully monitored.

Everything was going well until I suddenly heard the water boil over.

"Ssssss," went the steam. I reached over to take the pan off the burner, embarrassed that such an accomplished chef couldn't even boil water without it boiling over.

"Geeze," I said. It was no problem draining the water, putting in the butter, stirring in the powdered cheese, and mixing it all together. But the fact is I'd failed.

"Let me tell you why that happened," she said. "Short term memory is affected by strokes. So once you start something you're likely to forget about it due to the stroke. It's not your fault, it's just what happens. But we'll have to find ways to help you remember. Let's go back to the day room."

Connie had been waiting for me. But it wasn't until the drive home to Big Timber that I could share what happened. The gist of the conversation was simple. I thought I could speak; but I couldn't even find words that started with a letter as simple as "S." I thought I'd be able to copy a simple crossover step that any child could do, but I couldn't get the steps right. I knew for sure I knew what to do with a blue box of Kraft Macaroni and Cheese, but the water boiled over.

Speech therapy knew what its mission had to be.

Physical therapy knew what its mission had to be.

Occupational therapy knew what its mission had to be.

And slowly, but not yet by name, I knew what my mission had to be. Somehow I had to gain awareness. Somehow my assessment of the stroke had to change. And somehow I had to get my life back.

Headway was the place.

Life was the game. David, Chris, Carol, Mandi, and Nicole were the coaches.

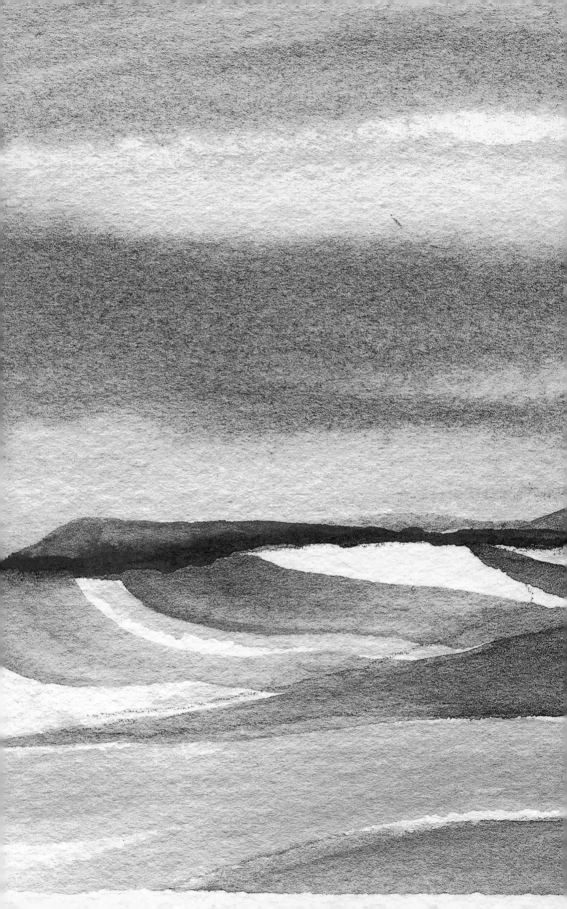

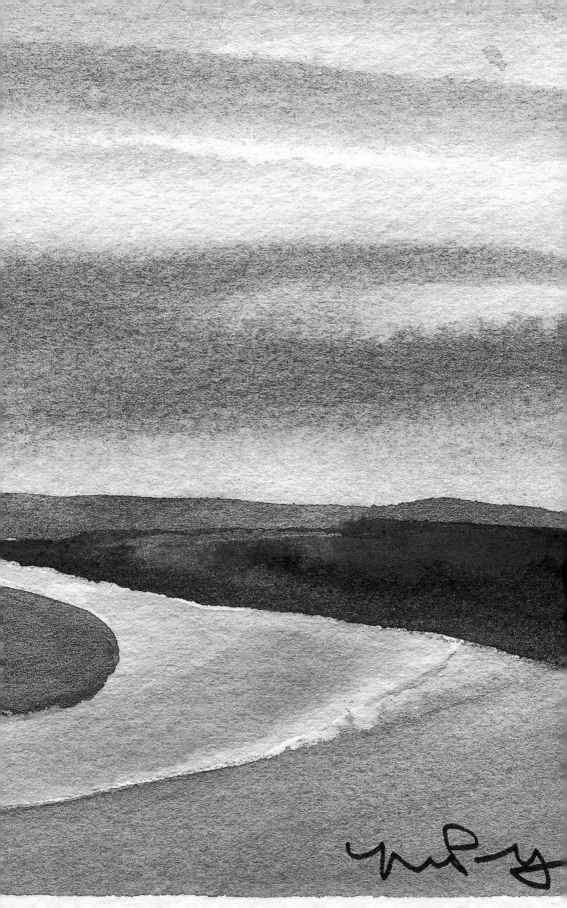

chapter eleven
beginnings are difficult

...

On a September morning in the fall of 1983, at Union Theological Seminary in New York City, I walked into a crowded classroom to begin studying the Old Testament. What I knew about Moses I owed to Sunday school and the miracle of cinema, but not much else. I had heard about the wisdom of Solomon, knew a few of the Psalms, could poetically affirm that God created heaven and earth, but that was about it. I had never regularly read the Bible or attended Bible studies. No matter, what I didn't know could be learned. I sat down and waited for the lecture to begin, figuring the first words would be, "In the beginning."

But that's not what she said.

"Beginnings are difficult," said Dr. Phyllis Trible, emphasizing each word as though it spoke volumes. She paused for a moment, having completely captured our attention and my imagination. Instead of beginning in chapter one, she began at the intersection of God's Word and human history.

"God said to Abram, 'Leave your country, your people and your father's household and go to the land I will show you.'" And then she repeated her first carefully chosen words: "Beginnings are difficult." They inevitably involve risking the unknown. They inevitably require risk, hope and courage. If we were to understand God, she seemed to be saying, we must also take a step. There would be time in the coming months to contemplate the creation stories in all their cosmic majesty. But our study began with history. First we were to join with Abram and pack our bags for a long journey.

It would be a full year before she lectured on the opening lines of Genesis. By then we traced the fitful rehabilitation of the torn and troubled world. Slavery gave way to a promised land. Voices of justice recoiled at the presence of injustice. Kings led, and then were led astray, words were heard, forgotten, remembered and then heeded in new ways. Throughout it all people made and called for new beginnings. Sometimes they did so of their own choosing. Sometimes events forced their hand. Either way, the three words of Dr. Trible's lecture proved themselves true:

Beginnings are difficult.

Although the "re" in rehabilitation implies a return to life -- the return of speech, the return of motion, the return of thought, the return of a job--there actually is no such thing as a complete return when the impairment is severe. Nor should there be. Abram's call was to move forward, not backward. Indeed, the consequences of moving backward are often disastrous. Jonah tried it and found himself in the belly of a whale; Lot's wife tried it and turned into a pillar of salt. Rehabilitation is actually about the habilitation of a new world. Life is not static. It moves. It changes. We adapt.

It is ironic and unfortunate that our impression of therapy often works against us just when we need it the most. There is something about the word that conjures visions of others guiding us back into life. We take a step, therapists make sure we don't fall, we take another step, and at the end of the day we're fixed. But the idea of a cure works against adaptation. Indeed, it even has the power to deny the theology of creation. Taken as a whole, the biblical story speaks of a God who seems to be better at responding to problems than preventing them in the first place. We were rescued from slavery and had to adapt as freedom came our way in a land of milk and honey. God did not stop Jonah from throwing himself into the sea, but did find a way to bring him both to his senses and to dry land. The idea that therapy is about new life instead of a nostalgic return to the past can't help but be abrasive. We would much prefer it if at the end of the day the therapists would say, "As you were" and we could return to life as it was. Instead they say, "This is a new day," emphasizing the word "new." Although I knew this in my mind, my heart resisted it.

Beginnings are difficult.

The chart on the Headway wall had me signed up for an hour of speech therapy; an hour of occupational therapy; an hour with a counselor named Mary, some physical therapy, a lunch break and an hour of Head Ed. Speech therapy came first.

I anticipated that speech therapy would both help me regain the gift of inflection and pick up the files the stroke had strewn across the floor of my mind. To my surprise, Chris did so by repairing the brain that controls speech. She called me over to the wooden table in the middle of the day room and handed me a piece of paper. An exercise that seemingly had nothing to do with speech had everything to do with speech.

"This is Simon Says," she said. The piece of paper had 19 lines of seemingly simple directions.

1. Print the words RELATIONAL DATABASE
2. Change the second vowel from each end to an S
3. Move the second vowel from the left to the immediate left of the second L from the left.
4. Delete the third consonant from the right.
5. Change the first L from the left to an F.
6. Move the second T from the left to the first place on the right.
7. Delete the sixth letter from the right.
8. Reverse the order of the first through third letters from the right.
9. Move the second vowel from the right to the immediate right of the second consonant from the left.
10. Insert an S in the first position on the left.
11. Delete the third vowel from the right.
12. Change the first T from the left to an M.
13. Exchange the positions of the fifth and sixth consonants from the left.
14. Move the middle vowel to the immediate right of the T.
15. Delete the seventh consonant from the right.
16. Move the second and third letters from the left to the immediate right of the O.
17. Change the D to a Y.
18. Delete the third vowel from the right;.
19. Delete every S.

"When you're done you'll have a recognizable word," she said. All I had to do was to follow the directions. And so I began. After each instruction I made sure I had done it correctly, but it soon became obvious my answers were headed nowhere. I erased and began again. To no avail the page filled with little arrows I had drawn indicating where the letters should go. On the 19th line I wrote: Orlelnybtoe…a word that certainly didn't look familiar.

I tried the exercise again.

And then again.

And then yet again, ending up with nonsense each and every time. As I worked Chris watched my progress, but also interacted with the other therapists who strolled through the day room on one assignment or another. At first the constant movement and the various conversations distracted. Didn't they know we were trying to concentrate? What kind of a teacher would carry on a conversation when her students were in the midst of an exam? No matter what I did, I couldn't filter out the sounds or follow the directions that promised to eventually lead to a coherent word. It is easy to think that therapy is something anyone can do, that it is made up of a somewhat random string of intense short-term assignments followed by fun and games. But actually there is a purpose for everything that happens. What I mistook for rudeness was actually part of the therapy. In both physical and cognitive therapy patients are asked to do a little more than they can do and a little less than magical thinking would have them do. The atmosphere of the day room was gently controlled chaos. If it became overwhelming one therapist or another would offer a kind word. One does not learn about the return to life in a vacuum.

"Why don't you take it home with you, and try it there?" Chris said.

"I don't know why I can't do it."

"Remember the file folders? They're all over the floor and until they're rearranged, it's going to be a challenge."

I saw a Scrabble game on the shelf and reached for it. Perhaps, if I used my hands and my arms, not just my brain, I could sequence the letters. I opened the box, found the letters and placed them in the wooden letter-rack. Sure enough, it did help. There was a way to solve the problem. Whenever I used the Scrabble board, I could figure things out. Whenever I relied on thoughts alone, I was utterly lost no matter how carefully I tried to get it right. It was all a matter of unlocking sequence.

We take sequence as a mark of intelligence for an individual and a mark of civilization for societies. Human beings are problem solvers. There is virtually no activity that does not involve sequence. To write a word one letter follows another until meaning is found. And then, that meaning links with another sequenced set of letters that make up the next word. The words are then sequenced as well until a meaningful sentence appears. Without sequence there is no meaning. Without sequence, problem solving, to say nothing of communication, is an elusive art.

"Why was sequence so difficult?" I later asked David.

"Well, the sequence part of your brain was damaged in the stroke. Normally sequence is a function of the left side of the brain, but the brain is remarkably interconnected, so what happens in one place can't help but affect other parts of the brain. Also I suspect that you used to learn not by following directions but by envisioning a problem's solution using the right side of your brain. Actually Einstein did that. He would actually imagine himself to be a light ray, for example. Then he would imagine what happens when gravity begins to bend the ray of light he's riding. I think you have gone through life in a similar way. You learned by imagining something and then wondering what happens when life intervenes. So when you lost so much of your right brain you also lost your capacity to solve problems as you'd always solved them before. Instead you had to suddenly use the left side of your brain, which is something you hadn't really relied on before. You were learning to learn again from the very beginning."

"Okay, let's take a break," Chris said.

I was only too glad to comply. Meanwhile a young woman in a wheelchair came into the room cackling with laughter. She had been teasing and playing tag with one of the therapists and was now trying to escape into the day room. They were clearly having a good time, but the sound, the sound, the sound was so sharp. I looked around the room to see if others were equally distracted, but they weren't. A young man named Paul sat on one of the light green Lazy Boy armchairs, dozing off to sleep. He held both forearms in front of him, as though their motion had been frozen in time. Another young woman took careful steps, and when she spoke her words were hard to discern. An older man who was an insurance agent before his accident looked healthy as a horse, but had suffered brain injury from a car accident. He rarely appeared without an armful of Aflac ducks, notepads or keychains, which he enjoyed giving away. The goal of his therapy was an eight word sentence: I'd like to go back to work again. His livelihood depended on it.

It was time for Head Ed. We gathered in a small semicircle in front of the schedule board. Dr. Gumm sat down in front of us, holding a model brain. The organ we know about, but rarely think about, was right there, in his hands, and Head Ed was a time to learn about it. The questions we asked that day were the questions we would be living with for the rest of our lives.

"Why is it we get so tired?" I asked.

"That's a common symptom of brain injury," said David.

"Is it because the remaining brain just isn't strong enough to carry the load?"

"You might say that," said David.

"How do we explain this to others?" one asked. "When they see me they say, 'You look so well!' Then I just don't know what to say."

"That's a real dilemma," said David. "You do look just fine, but that's because they cannot see what happened to your brain or how different your life really is. There is such a lack of understanding about brain injury. Insurance companies don't get it; friends don't easily understand it, employers have a very hard time taking it into consideration."

"I just can't remember anything," said Jerry. "I have all these clients. I'm their agent, but its like I just can't keep up with it all. I'll forget to return a call, and no matter how many notes I make it's like I don't know what to do. I get so tired that I just can't put in a full day." His wife nodded her head.

"And what happened to you?" asked David. He knew, of course, but the question prompted us to tell our stories.

"I had a car accident," said Jerry. He added that accidents were nothing new. He even brought a picture of the airplane crash he had survived years earlier.

"You know brain injury is cumulative," said David. "Injuries we have when we're 14 years old or so stay with us, so when there is an accident later in life its impact is compounded. That's part of the reason wearing helmets is so important, and is maybe why I just can't watch boxing. Every punch to the head hurts the brain, and when that happens over and over again the injury is severe."

Speaking slowly, also in a monotone, Paul shared his story. He had been run over not once, but twice, in the same accident, and taken to the emergency room where he lay in a coma for weeks before waking up only to find he could not walk, that his arms were seemingly frozen in place, that he had lost all taste. It was a "hit and run" accident and the driver had not yet been found. Extensive surgeries had saved his life, but his future looked bleak.

The young woman in the wheelchair shared her story. She and her infant daughter were at a stoplight when a truck behind her failed to slow down and rammed into her at full speed. She was also taken to the hospital where she fell into a coma. During the coma she could not have known that her daughter was killed instantly in the accident.

David talked a bit about comas, and how fortunate a person is when he or she can emerge from the deep sleep. Years ago it was thought best to not interfere with the brain when its swelling induced a coma. But now most hospitals recognize that relieving the pressure in the brain is essential if the patient is to survive. A hole is drilled, a catheter inserted and pressure relieved. Then life can begin anew as billions of remaining neurons regroup. To hear the stories of the other patients was heartening and heart-breaking. It established a depth of connection that became therapeutic in its own right. We cared about each other's progress and noted each other's outlook.

"We'll meet again on Thursday," said David. To learn to live with our brains we needed to learn about our brains, so Head Ed met twice a week.

I looked at the schedule board. We had an hour for lunch and then the square alongside my name on the board said "Occupational Therapy." Connie and I went to the cafeteria and then returned to the day room and waited for one o'clock.

One of the OT therapists, Catherine, called me over to her table and handed me a small piece of paper. "What I'd like you to do is to go up to the pharmacy and find the price for each of these items. If you can't find them ask the pharmacist." There were no curve balls on the list. All I needed to do was report on the price of a bottle of aspirin, a bottle of Tylenol, a box of bandages and a bottle of antiseptic. The pharmacy was right inside the front door of the building. It was a hospital pharmacy with an aura of intentional medicine. There were no Star magazines, no rows of peanuts or aisles of greeting cards. Actually it had very few shelves. For some reason I assumed the prices would be far more than those at Cole's drug in Big Timber.

"Okay," I said, taking the list and heading out of the dayroom. The elevator was exactly where it was supposed to be, and so was the pharmacy. I began to look over the shelves in search of the various items Catherine asked me to find. I looked high; I looked low; to no avail.

"May I help you?" asked one of the pharmacists.

"I'm looking for a bottle of aspirin."

"It's on that shelf," she said, pointing to the shelf behind me. And sure enough there was a bottle of aspirin. But it didn't have a price tag on it. I would have to ask how much it cost. Suddenly the sheer lunacy of the exercise overwhelmed me. Nothing depended on the price of those aspirin tablets. A war raged in Iraq, a church wondered what its future held, colleagues all over the country were working their heart out to bring together the world of faith and health and I was checking out the price of a bottle of aspirin. A woman made her way to the counter and handed over a prescription. The pharmacist perused it carefully, and they had a brief discussion about the side affects of the drug. I imagined it must be a cancer drug or an inhaler upon which life itself depended. The purchase mattered. Finally, it was my turn.

"How much is this bottle?"

"Two twenty-nine," came the answer. I wrote down the number, wadded up the paper and went back downstairs completely ashamed.

It was time to go home. We walked out to the car. Connie got into the driver's seat, I opened the passenger door and got in. Normally when we drove the sequence was reversed. But driving was still forbidden. All day long I had failed at elementary lessons. Frustration boiled over.

"I'm not going back," I said, my words brimming over with anger. "What's the point of this?"

"So, you're not going back," she said.

"No."

"So you can't do the puzzles but you can make a decision to stop therapy?"

She needed to say no more. We both knew the next day therapy would begin again and that one way or another I'd be there. When Connie didn't have the strength to drive me people from the church would volunteer. Sometimes they had errands to run in Billings. For the most part Big Timber adhered to rural socialism in which residents go out of their way to support local business establishments, even if the prices are a bit more. But there is often a corresponding urge to run errands in the big city. I loved the conversations we had along the way to Billings. We would talk about all manner of things. I would try to describe therapy, or try to describe how it felt to not feel like oneself. They were always encouraging, always gentle, always full of life. One morning a rancher offered to drive me to Billings. I had baptized his two children in the creek that runs through their ranch. We were about half way to town when his cell phone rang. Calving season had begun, and one cow was having difficulty with the birth of her calf. He and Bret, his 14 year-old son, had been keeping a careful eye on it all night long. As labor progressed Bret called to give a report. He had stayed home from school to be with the cow. Remy gave some suggestions, saying that he would be back in just a few hours.

"Can you manage?"

"Yes."

"Well, keep an eye on her. I'll be there as soon as I can." A wave of guilt ran through me. He had left the ranch to take me to the hospital where I'd be working on brain teasers. Between an elementary school puzzle and the well-being of a cow and its calf, cognitive therapy didn't hold much weight.

"I'm sorry," I said. "It's all right," Remy reassured me. "They'll make it okay." Bret knew what to do. It turned out that the cow and its calf made it just fine.

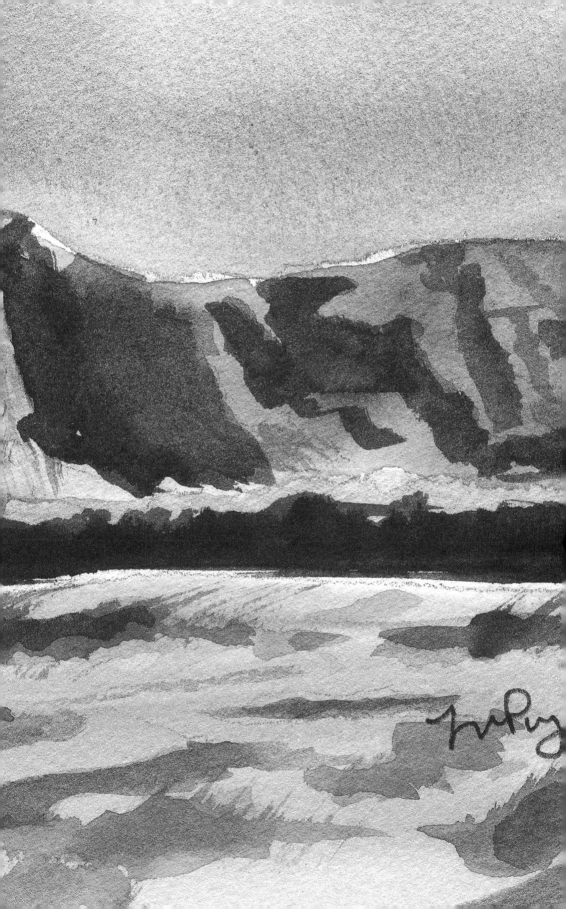

chapter twelve
the book

* * *

The beige metal bookcase in the Headway day room held the rudiments of a small library. Compared to the cupboards that were full of therapeutic games, the bookshelf was not very well tended. It almost seemed to be an afterthought. One afternoon, between therapy sessions, I went over and browsed through the dozen or so books and journals that leaned up against each other in haphazard fashion. Most of the covers were as academic as their corresponding text. But one caught my eye.

The book's title was *Awareness of Deficit After Brain Injury: Clinical and Theoretical Issues,* edited by George P. Prigatano and Daniel L. Schacter.[8] On the cover there was a rudimentary drawing of a face. It appeared to be a woman's face, but I couldn't be sure. Either way, its thin and somewhat fearful lines had been drawn by an uncertain hand. Curiously enough, the right half of the forehead was completely missing. In its place were the words:

I am a normal person

with part of my head

off in never never land.

(Will I ever retrieve it?)

The words could not have been written by a child. Children don't use the word "retrieve." Because the left side was missing I knew the person had experienced a right brain stroke. The startling drawing and caption made me curious. David and I had talked about anosognosia; here was a book about it. The picture had to represent an extreme case, I said to myself. I wasn't anywhere near as severe as the person who drew such a strange picture with its probing

---

8 *Awareness of Deficit After Brain Injury: Clinical and Theoretical Issues*, edited by George P. Prigatano and Daniel L. Schacter, Oxford University Press, New York, 1991.

•

question. Nevertheless I began to thumb through the book. It didn't take long to see it had not been written for the general public. One sentence read, "Implicit in the idea of an intimate association of anosognosia with general confusion or intellectual deterioration is the temptation to explain away anosognosia as one aspect of a global, undifferentiated disorder of cognitive function." The end of each chapter cited 20 or 30 references drawn from all manner of professional journals such as the *Archives of Neurology, Neuropsychologia,* and *Neurosurgery.*

I leafed through the pages looking for pictures. One MRI looked vaguely familiar. Most of the brain tissue was gray, just as it should have been. But one portion showed a small white river flowing into the gray sea surrounding it. The caption indicated the picture showed where a tumor had been surgically removed. The patient's name was "R." I began to read about "R." Unhindered by neurological jargon, her story emerged as one paragraph led to the next.

"Seizure activity in a highly educated and successful professional businesswoman led to the discovery of a right frontal astrocytoma that was surgically removed. The patient returned to work one year after the operation but at a much reduced work load. She originally denied having any problems. However, at the insistence of her spouse she eventually was referred for neuropsychological assessment. At that time she verbally accepted her 'deficits.'"

"Neuropsychological examination revealed excellent abilities. There were minor exceptions: left-sided motor slowing; perseverance on the California Verbal Learning Test; tangentiality in conversation; mild distractibility; and mild difficulty on certain attentional tasks." The words hit home. I too was easily distracted; I too had a hard time staying with a conversation. I always wanted to add something else or change horses midstream.

"Her daily life, however, was characterized by (as the patient herself stated) 'all standard frontal lobe signs.' She had difficulty getting up, showering, dressing, and getting to work before 11:00 a.m. She would forget to perform even minor daily tasks. In these and other regards, her husband stated that she was a different individual."

She had changed and didn't realize it. That's what I too had been told. I read her husband's words over and over again. "She was a different individual." I suspected it wasn't just a matter of being unable to start the morning, unable to give ideas traction, unable to make decisions, unable to remember the grocery list. All of those are understandable, forgivable, and all are of secondary importance. Everyone forgets why they went to the store. But her husband wasn't talking about accidental forgetfulness. He had probably lived with that for years, and teased her about it endlessly, as most couples do. No...he was addressing something entirely different. She was now a different individual. She was now <u>disabled</u>. Something had to be done and she agreed to begin therapy, just as I had agreed to enter therapy.

"Because of her generally excellent results on testing and her high level of prior functioning, rehabilitation was initiated. The following methods were attempted: use of verbal self-regulation to guide behavior; training in the focusing of attention; practice in establishing appropriate goals and monitoring behavior; and increasing the awareness of her problems and the level of functioning, of which she was now capable. Rehabilitation over 18 months had limited success. Signs in her office ("stay on task") and verbal self-regulation ("I will finish this one job first") did improve work productivity and punctuality in daily life, but only to a certain limit.

"At weekly sessions, with therapeutic guidance, appropriate employment goals were established for the following week. Charting the success of achieving these goals attempted to increase her awareness of actual functioning in relation to expected functioning. This objective feedback revealed her lack of success. Even though her stated goals were significantly less than her previous functioning level, her maximum achievement was only 50 percent of the stated goals. In addition, formal feedback from both her employer and her subordinates was on one occasion so devastating and personal that she was crestfallen. By the next session, however, the implications of this review appeared to have minimal impact on her decisions concerning her work."

I realized in an instant that, for her, the jig was up. She had changed. She didn't realize it. But her employer did. They were going to ease her out. The next paragraph confirmed my suspicions.

"Total or partial disability appeared to be a logical conclusion. It would enable her to enjoy her family, obtain a reasonable pension, and possibly find less demanding alternative employment. The patient accepted this decision. During the final therapy meeting, however, the intellectual acceptance of her limitations was abrogated with the verbalization that she could and would return to her previous level of functioning within one year."

Once again the words hit home. We want rehabilitation to be restoration. Instead it turns out to be an epic struggle. Not surprisingly it is found in ancient texts. One night on the verge of meeting up with his brother Esau, from whom he had stolen a blessing, Jacob fell asleep and wrestled with a creature that would not let him go. All night long they fought. Finally the dawn broke, and Jacob received both a limp and a blessing. He would never be the person he was. Instead he was given a new name, Israel. What happened to Jacob, happens to us as we too find a new identity.

In one of our meetings, Mary, my social worker took the battle to heart and asked me a simple question.

"What would you say to a parishioner if one of them had a stroke? Would you counsel anger?"

"Of course not," I said.

"Wouldn't you ask them to adapt?"

"Of course I would," I said. "I would say that acceptance isn't easy but eventually it is necessary. And I would probably add that there is a reason for them to live, that their life had not yet come to an end."

"Well?" she gently said.

"I know."

"Do you?"

"No."

R's therapists tried everything to make her come to terms with a new reality.

"Role playing was used to evaluate her awareness (knowledge) of her situation and the appropriate steps to take to remedy it. Acting as her own direct supervisor, she analyzed the facts and made appropriate recommendations concerning her own employment as well as her daily life: continuation of her loss of privilege to drive a car; based on her work performance and medical condition, obtainment of a disability pension; and presentation of practical steps to investigate the best type of pension. When asked, she stated that these conclusions were logical based on the evidence. Once removed from her role-playing position, however, she was no longer able to make the same judgments in relation to her real-life personal situation and was determined to return to work at her pre-surgery level of functioning.

"Several observations may be made concerning this case study," the book continued. No kidding, I thought. "She was, in many respects, totally 'normal' or unimpaired. Not only did she exhibit no disturbance in most abilities tested, her test performance was often superior. Even supposed 'frontal lobe' tests were often unimpaired, likely reflecting her superior intelligence. Although at the time she actively denied or minimized problems, most often she acknowledged the deficit. She did not appear to be unaware (in the sense of lacking knowledge) or indeed totally unconcerned, evidenced by her desire to continue therapy to improve. The most significant disturbance occurred in one aspect of self-awareness; the use of the knowledge she possessed in relation to decisions about her future."

I closed the book and put it back on the shelf. The question written where the forehead should be on the book's cover touched both hope and despair of heart and mind:

"I am a normal person with part of my head off in never never land. Will I ever retrieve it?"

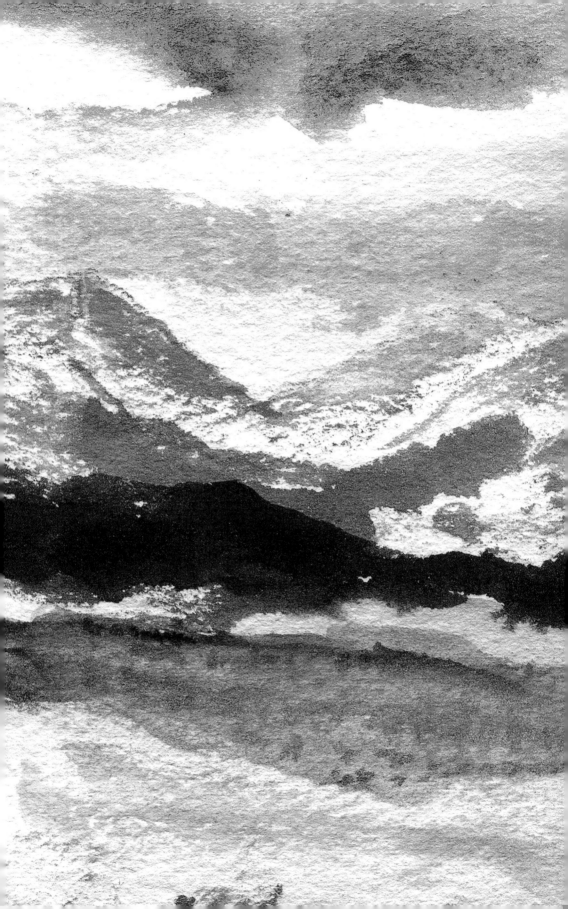

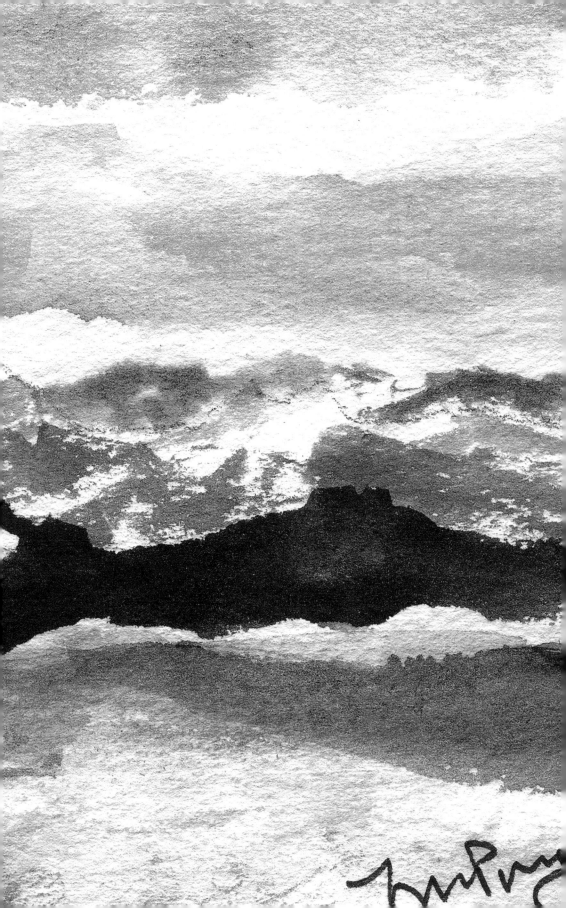

chapter thirteen
the placeholder's conversation

•••

March could not be held at bay. Winter had spoken and spring seemed years
away. The church had been prayerful, patient and kind beyond all expectation. I
once heard a story about "placeholding." When someone leaves home, he or she
selects a placeholder. That person makes a place in his or her heart for the one
who will be away. Everyone knows that one way or another there will be a day of
return, however brief it might be. When that day comes there will be many
stories to share. "Where have you been? What have you learned?" It would not
be an idle conversation. Truth would hold the floor and life would be the speaker.

The church had been my placeholder and I, in turn, held a place for them in
the season of being away. Nearly four months had passed since the 11th of
November. It was time to assess where we had been and what the future would
hold. Connie and I chose an evening and invited the pastoral care committee and
a number of deacons whose presence we valued and trusted over to our home.
For years we had held most of our diaconate meetings in the living room rather
than at church. Hospitality is a form of worship, and these get-togethers gave us
as chance to break bread together while trying to discern where God was taking
us. In the course of an afternoon meeting someone would say, "Good idea, Larry,
but give us a break!" and then they would come up with a much better idea I
wouldn't have considered in a million years. We enjoyed the pleasure of each
other's company.

As each one arrived, a wave of emotion ran through me. Byron came in first,
then Kirby; then Barbara. It was around her kitchen table that I first learned
about the First Congregational Church in Big Timber, Montana. She is one of the

few people I've ever heard say, "I like committees. That's how you get things done." Sox was there. He ran the lumber company his grandfather had founded nearly a century before. His loving presence was always steady, thoughtful and generous in spirit. Tom, the church moderator, came in. A carpenter and contractor whose buildings reflected both structural and spiritual integrity, his care for the congregation during my absence ran as deep as the still waters that restore the soul. With him was Shirle, his wife, a paralegal and artist who lovingly enlisted every child in the entire Sunday school to make a stunning quilt that adorned and inspired the sanctuary. And, of course, Connie.

We greeted them, asked if they wanted a cup of coffee, and formed a circle in the living room. I thanked them for coming, realizing as I spoke how odd it was that this was our first meeting as a group since the stroke. Logic told me that I had been irresponsible, just letting things slide from day to day. Perhaps I had been waiting for the three months to pass. Or perhaps I had been wary of a meeting in which there were more than one or two people. Whatever the reason, the facts spoke for themselves. It was our first formal meeting.

We opened in prayer. I shared with them how grateful I was to be alive, thanked them for their prayers, shared the story of therapy and the progress I'd been making.

During or after illness it is always a challenge to know what should be said when someone asks, "How are you?" Too much detail sounds like complaint or a prelude to hypochondria. Not enough detail sounds like a brush-off. And so we develop litanies that pass for truth without naming it. Mine were, "I've lost some cells, maybe a billion or so, but it's getting better and I'm beginning to feel like myself again; I miss words, but not as many as I did; Therapy is hard work but it's great." I took care to not miss my words, to make sure each came out correctly. Such litanies tend to be self-serving. They rarely pass the placeholder test that calls for genuine conversation. Everyone in the room had already heard the litanies. And everyone knew there was more to be said.

And then I made the heroic pitch.

"The doctors said I could not go back to work for three months. Four months have just about passed. I know what I can do and I know what I can't do.

Knowing those two things I am sure I can return to work. It is time to begin again. I know I can do it and I am sure we can find a way."

When hope wraps itself in the heroic one must be careful lest it deny the truth. Overcoming the odds is inevitably heroic, universally esteemed, and a publicly traded commodity. Industries and fund-raisers launch heroic wars on cancer, MS, or heart disease. Such wars are both acceptable and hard to criticize. Who could be against a cure? But they can also be an exercise in denial. The implications of anosognosia never crossed my mind as I made the case for return. My failure to mention anosognosia only confirmed its strange power to hide reality. A look of concern crossed their faces as they instinctively discerned the difference between hope and wishful thinking, the difference between hope and expectation. Which was it? We mulled it over for a few minutes. In my mind I knew that if it could be done, we would find a way to do it. I would adjust; they would adjust; we would continue in ministry. We knew how to do that.

We paused for a moment. And then a placeholder conversation began.

"I need to speak," Connie said, her voice laden with emotion. In her hands she held the large folder with the MRI negatives. In her heart was the depth of courage and compassion that truth requires.

"I want you to see these to understand what we're dealing with," she said. She stood up and so did everyone else. She took the films out of their folder and held them up in front of one of the lamps. As she did everyone moved a step or two closer. There they were: my skull, the gray brain tissue on the left side of the skull; and the lifeless ice shelf on the right side of the image.

"He thinks he can go back but he doesn't know how badly he was hurt," Connie said. "It's not that he doesn't want to; he can't. Those cells are gone. I know he wants to go back, and I know you want him back, but look at this."

The group was as astonished as we were when we first saw the MRI. Slowly they returned to their seats and our small circle reformed. Truth can never steal hope but it can trump false expectation.

It was Kirby's turn to speak.

"She's right," he said. "It is a miracle he lived through this stroke. Honestly, when we look at what you've just seen we have no idea why he isn't in a nursing home or how he survived. I'm really concerned that he is still fragile, certainly more fragile than he realizes." Spiritually Kirby knew I had to let go if life was to have a chance. So did Tom, the moderator. Several weeks earlier we had shared a Bible study in which Jesus asked the disciples to cast their nets in another direction. To the disciples it seemed a foolish request. But they obeyed and brought in a far greater catch than anyone could have imagined. Would I cast my nets in another direction? Would it be a forced option? Would I be willing, and able, to give up the confines of "I want my life back" and yield to a new creation? Rhetorical questions seldom provide traction but they can often spark rebellion. A flood of thoughts passed through me as my expectations for the meeting disintegrated. After all, therapy was the hardest work I'd ever done in my life, didn't that mean I was capable of working? Couldn't we try a return to ministry and see how it went? In another month or two everything might be just fine.

"He doesn't understand," Connie said with tears in her eyes. "The cells he needs to understand aren't there."

I suddenly felt surrounded. This wasn't the way the meeting was supposed to go. There was no way to escape the MRI's message or the placeholder conversation. I wish that I had thanked Connie for the depth of her love and the courage it took for her to speak. I wish I had thanked Kirby for his healing ministry and Tom for the net he helped Scripture cast our way. I wish I had said something gentle, like "Let's give it a bit more time. Therapy runs for a few more weeks, and if I rest the healing can't help but continue." But that is not what I said. Instead an image leaped into my mind. I had seen the film *Old Yeller* when I was a child. Old Yeller was a yellow lab in the Lassie tradition. His family loved him and he loved them with the unquestioned loyalty dogs have for their owners. But when he contracted rabies they had no choice but to put him down. Both the dog and the family were caught by a set of circumstances neither had asked for. The scene of the young boy taking the shotgun while fighting back tears made Old Yeller a film of unforgettable pathos.

I looked around the room.

"What are we going to do, shoot old Yeller?" I asked.

The words astonished me. They were utterly out of character and lacking in judgment, to say nothing of wisdom. I'm sure they astonished everyone in the room as well. One telltale sign of a right-brain stroke is that everything appears just fine for a moment, but extend the conversation, and its symptoms come into view. A brain without brakes is not given to nuance. The measured pastor, whose life had been one of balancing emotions both in his life and in the lives of others, was nowhere to be found. The pastor who preached a Gospel of hope fought for denial instead.

"No," they all said with a kindness and concern I will never forget. "That's not what we're saying."

"I'm sorry," I said. "I didn't mean that."

"We know," they said with consummate compassion and grace.

"Then we should take steps to get an interim minister for a while," I said. I knew who it had to be. I didn't want someone who would come in to change everything we had worked so lovingly to create. We needed a placeholder until I could return. We needed someone who would love people; who would minister in a time of grief; who had the voice of experience. That would be Ray Schatz. I had known Ray for a number of years and had seen him serve in interim ministries. The next morning we called and made the arrangements.

The meeting drew to a close. We said a prayer. My friends walked out into the night. Connie and I embraced in the light of truth without illusion. Neither of us could have known a new ice shelf was about to break loose.

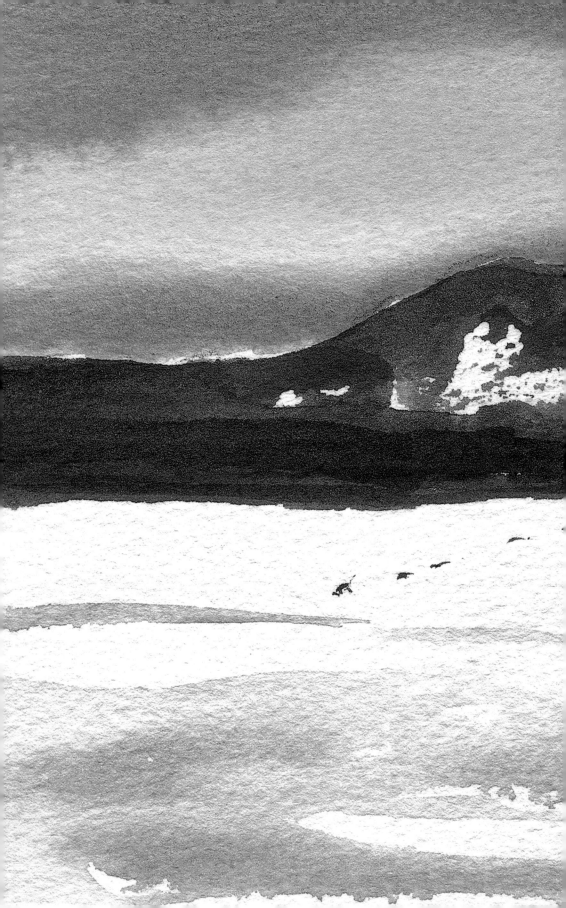

chapter fourteen
incoherence

...

We set a Sunday to share with the church that there would have to be yet more time before I could return. It was a service I wanted to lead. In January we had arranged for a guest pastor to share a service with me. He would do the sermon, I would lead the prayers and give the benediction. His sermon was excellent, his kindness genuine, his concern authentic. But for me the service was disorienting and a bit frightening. When it was time to sing I could not find the note and an off-tune groan emerged before I could step away from the microphone. With both of us in the pulpit, my inability to understand spatial relationships caught up with me. I did not know where to stand, and sitting felt awkward. Fitting into an external scheme was perplexing and emotionally devastating. I knew that pulpit, those people, the windows, the hymnals, the service, but I could not connect with any of it. Ministry is all about sharing, but sharing is about relationship, and I could not find my bearings. And so on this March Sunday I needed to give the sermon and lead the service. When one cannot fit in the only option is to lead and hope for the best. The only addition to the service would be a word from Kirby who would sit with the congregation and then come forward. I was grateful for whatever he said. When a man looks just fine, but says he must leave because of illness, it can't help but be confusing. His words would give a sense of clarity to anosognosia's coup.

The service was pregnant with emotion. We centered ourselves for worship, sang an opening hymn, thanked God for life, prayed for others and asked for guidance in our own lives. When the time came for the children's sermon they came forward, full of life, and sat on the two front steps of our beautiful sanctuary. They had not seen me for four months; and I had not seen them. I told them how much I had missed them and that I had to stay away for yet another period of time. I told them I would miss them but would be back, and then watched them leave the sanctuary and head for their Sunday School classes. It was time for Kirby to address the congregation. He acknowledged that he had to play the "bad guy" and that it was an uncomfortable role for him. But he minced no words as he spoke with characteristic concern.

"Larry is not yet ready to come back," he said. "I know he wants to, and I know we want him to come back. But his life is at risk. If he does not take time to rest he may not live out the month. It really is a matter of life and death for him. I don't like saying that, but it is the truth."

We finished the service with the benediction we used every Sunday:

"Go now, into a torn and troubled world, and be of good cheer. Comfort the afflicted, strengthen the faint-hearted, render to no one evil for evil, no matter how tempting it may and will most certainly seem, and know in the depth of your soul that you are loved and called by God this day and forevermore."

And then, we sang the blessing song: May the Lord; mighty God, bless you and keep you forever. Grant you peace, perfect peace, courage in every endeavor. Lift up your eyes and see God's face, and God's grace, forever. May the Lord, mighty God, bless and keep you forever." We wiped away a few tears, greeted each other and went downstairs for a Norsk cup of coffee.

It was time to go home.

Monday morning came with its usual rhythm. I awoke, went downstairs, glanced at the newspaper to see if it made sense, and started my workout on the Nordic Track. I listened to NPR's "Morning Edition" knowing that each news segment was about five minutes and that the 90-second naturalist did indeed last exactly 90 seconds. Before long the 20 minutes had passed; I moved to the free weights; did some rudimentary Tai Chi and then headed upstairs for a shower. After dressing I walked downstairs to the kitchen to test my blood sugar. The test isn't hard to do. One simply pricks the end of a finger with a lancet, squeezes out a drop of blood and applies it to a test strip. Not surprisingly, I usually chose a finger on my nerve-deadened left hand. It only takes five seconds for the meter to give a reading. Then it was a simple matter of entering that number into my insulin pump, and hitting the ACTIVATE button to infuse a computer-determined dose.

And so, as I had thousands of times before, I walked through the kitchen, past the white refrigerator, past the stove and the blue Shaker cupboards and went over to the small drawer that held my testing equipment and my insulin supplies. I pricked my finger, gathered the drop of blood, and applied it to the strip. As I waited for the reading a strange feeling swept through me. It was faintly dizzying, faintly disconnecting. Something was happening to me. I looked at the numbers. They made no sense. I knew I had to do something with the pump according to those numbers but had no idea what, as numbers and meters floated in a miasma of confusion. Nothing made sense. How strange, I thought. Connie was in the living room reading a book. I was going to have to ask her for help. The notion almost brought a laugh to my lips. I walked over to her, still wondering how I could be so confused, and still half amused that I needed help. The words formed themselves in my mind before I spoke.

"Connie, I'm going to need some help," I would say. The words could not have been simpler.

"I need some help," I began to say. But to my utter astonishment a language I had never heard before came streaming out of my mouth. They were words, perhaps, but words I had never heard before that poured forth in a torrent of sound. Sometimes they came in a single phrase as the sounds repeated themselves, sometimes they shifted gears to make way for new sounds that constituted a language I had never spoken. Some words sounded as though they'd like to be Hawaiian, or Swahili, Sesotho, Crow, or perhaps Finnish. The torrent of undecipherable words all flowed from a single thought: "I need help." Had a Pentecostal believer been present he or she would have said I was praising God in ecstatic tongues. Perhaps so, but there was nothing more behind the words than a simple four-word sentence.

"I need some help," my mind said, in fluent English. There was nothing complicated about it. But I could not articulate even one of the words. "Lala manala mashi ki somai" I said. I could scarcely believe what I was hearing. And so I stopped, and then tried once again to say what needed to be said.

"I need some help." Once again an unrecognizable torrent of words spewed forth. They came without fear and as though they expected to be understood. They came with a certain bewilderment, perhaps wondering why Connie could not understand them. Although for years I had teased her and the kids by making up pretend languages that sounded remarkably coherent, she knew in an instant that I was not joking around. She ran to the phone and called the hospital, which was right across the street.

"Come on, we're going," she said. She reached out to steady me, even though my balance was just fine. "Of course that's what we will do," I said to myself in perfect English. I asked her about my blood sugar. It was a rational, important question. But once again the stream of glossolalia spewed forth. We went out to the car. She reached for the keys. I had them. I told her I had them but did not do so in English. Nickie was at the desk. She greeted us, and saw that I was walking. Everything looked just fine. I began to speak with her.

"Nicki, something's wrong," my mind said.

"Kalamasha mashiko, koshimano, seya ka chinso," my words said. I saw concern cross her face. Nurses came running and led me into the emergency room. They asked me to lay down on one of its two beds. As I lay down I kept talking, the words still streaming forth in a torrent of unintelligible sounds. Connie was there with me. When I saw someone I kept trying to say their name, but every attempt led to nothing but incoherence. By now my mild amusement gave way to apprehension. Everyone tried to calm me down. I trusted them and knew them by name but it was obvious nobody knew what to do, and that perhaps there was nothing to be done.

During my first stroke Tim, our oldest son, caught the first flight from Los Angeles to Billings. Ben flew in from Alaska. Emily came in from Minneapolis. Each of them surrounded me with love and care. Ben's twin brother, Andy, was working for a television station in Cheyenne, Wyoming, and could not leave his job. It suddenly occurred to me that I might die without having seen him, and so I kept trying to say his name over, and over again. The staff kept encouraging me to settle down as if the "event" would pass of its own accord. I tried to say "Tim," and even though a strange word emerged, I knew exactly who I was calling. I kept trying to say, "Ben, Emily, and Andy," to pull them closer as well. It is often said that one reaches out to loved ones when life slips away. I know this to be true. In those chaotic moments I kept trying to say the names of the children over and over again, trying to draw them close, wanting to reach out to them and to Connie. When the day comes that I do pass away, I know they will be drawn close to my soul.

I looked over and saw Connie standing with Kirby at the door of the emergency room. It was clear that the attack of aphasia confused him as much as it did me. Aphasia is a language disorder that results from damage to the parts of the brain responsible for speech. It can affect both speaking and understanding. I had known it as missing and mispronouncing single words. This fluent aphasia was something new. Connie kept saying, "It's a stroke. It's another stroke." He was reluctant to make the diagnosis. Perhaps it was just a TIA, transient ischemic attack, that would pass on its own in just a few minutes. TIAs are warning signs of an impending stroke but cause no lasting damage in and of themselves. And, of course, there was a third possibility. Perhaps it was an emotional breakdown. After all, glossolalia is a symptom of a mental disorder. Against my will I had just bid farewell to the church I loved and the ministry that gave me life. If it was simply stress then what I needed was rest. They administered a sedative and I surrendered to its slow collapse. Throughout it all the hospital staff was confused, concerned, and a bit scared. It was the first time they had experienced such a condition. They wheeled me out of the emergency room and into the hospital section of the clinic. Over the next few hours English began its slow return, as nonsense gave it a place or two in a line of speech. I quickly fell asleep and scarcely woke up for the next 24 hours. I stayed in the hospital for two full days. Finally English once again asserted its rightful presence as the beautiful language it is and aphasia returned to the hidden land in which it lives.

Convinced it was a stroke, Connie insisted on a consult with a neurologist in Billings. The neurology staff attributed it to a TIA and none of them seemed to think that an MRI was necessary. But Connie can be a very persistent woman and she finally persuaded Kirby to authorize an MRI. We went into Billings and to the MRI center that the two hospitals uneasily shared. The receptionist said, "Hi, Larry!" She looked familiar, but I could not place her name.

"It's Mandy," she said. I still could not place her. "You married us!" she said. Then I remembered. It was good to see her. Pastors always wonder how life will go for couples they marry. I could tell that things were going well; was glad they were still together, that their marriage had been meaningful and that their job with a mine in Wyoming had migrated to Montana. She took the requisite paperwork; showed me where to change my clothes for the MRI, and where to wait. I had been in that room before, and remembered leafing through its books to try and learn what strokes were all about.

The MRI took just a few minutes. When it was over I walked back up to Headway for the day's therapy session. I shared with the therapists what had happened, and they all said it sounded like a TIA. It had to be that because the aphasia didn't last. That afternoon my thinking was slow, my capacity to solve the problems virtually nil and I appeared tired to the staff. But scary though the aphasia had been, there didn't appear to be any permanent damage. The therapists all treated me with compassion. After all, something had happened to one of their patients. One can be a physician without establishing a relationship with a patient. I never saw the "king" after our original encounter, and he never sent a note or called to check in on the course of events after November 11th. It isn't relationship that reads X-rays, that gives the diagnoses; it is pure scientific data. In technology-driven medicine a caring doctor is nice but not necessary. But those who choose rehabilitation have a different take on healing. They know that building a relationship is absolutely essential. For months they hold the future of a patient in their hands and anything that jeopardizes that future affects them a great deal. It is no wonder love is often used to characterize their healing presence.

My therapy for the afternoon couldn't have been simpler. A new therapist handed me a sheet of paper that had a row of subtraction problems. All I had to do was solve them. The problems were not difficult. Any third grader could solve them. The therapist watched me slide the problem sheet front and center. I didn't know her name, but had seen her walk through the day room several times.

Perhaps it was Sonja. I looked over the problems and picked up the pencil.

$$
\begin{array}{ccc}
96 & 34 & 83 \\
\underline{-58} & \underline{-18} & \underline{-74}
\end{array}
$$

No problem, I thought to myself, but you can't take eight away from four, it's too big. You have to do something first. You have to borrow. You borrow from the three so then you have fourteen take away eight. What would that be? But I still saw the eight beneath the four. You can't take eight away from four. I crossed out the three to make it a two. But wouldn't that make it a twenty? How is that possible? But if I did that was it really a twenty, and I couldn't remember where the two would go, would it join up with the fourteen? A litany of subtraction rules ran though my mind to no avail. I stared at the problem again and crossed out numbers as though my incoherent marks might solve the problem. They didn't. I had no clue how to borrow. A third grader's math problem was incomprehensible.

Tears welled up within me. It was the first and only time in therapy that ever happened. I put my forehead on the table and began to quietly sob. Sonia stood up from her chair and gently placed her hand on my shoulder.

"It's okay," she said in a voice that was a perfect mixture of compassion, therapeutic insight and encouragement.

"We can come back to these. It will come back." I pushed the tears back, not knowing what else to do. As I did the memory of a story from seventh grade English class surfaced.

Once a week, on Friday afternoon, our seventh-grade English teacher at Euclid Junior High School read a story to us. She only read stories that she loved, and she read them giving each word, each sentence, the full emotion it deserved. Yes, we were Friday-afternoon restless on that September afternoon. Yes, our imaginations were pleasingly distracted by the astonishing beauty of the girl sitting in the desk just behind us, or along side us, or up there in the front row. And yet, when Mrs. Hewitt began reading we were entranced by her love of a well-written story. One Friday the story was entitled *Flowers for Algernon*. It concerned an ordinary mouse that had been given an experimental medication that transformed him into a genius. Algernon's keeper was a developmentally disabled man named Charlie. Given his limitations, he could care for mice, but that was about it. He was often tricked, shamed and taken advantage of by others who enjoyed teasing him as he cleaned the bathrooms. The scientists noticed that the medication made Algernon uncannily adept at running the mazes that once confused him. He could suddenly figure out whatever obstacle the lab placed in his way. They decided that if Algernon could benefit from the medication, Charlie might get smarter as well.

And it worked. Suddenly the man whose "friends" had been taking advantage of him could run circles around them. As Charlie came into his own, those who had been teasing him were shown to be what they really were—cruel, shallow and single dimensional people. As he progressed they regressed. But then, one day, Charlie noticed that Algernon inexplicably missed a turn in the maze he had previously mastered. The next day, the same thing happened. He again missed a turn and didn't know what to do. A week later he missed not one turn but two, and then three. Algernon's capacity and ability were both slipping away.

Charlie knew from Algernon's collapse that the handwriting was on the wall. He, too, would begin to decline. All that had been gained would be lost. He would soon be mopping the floors and laughing at the taunts thrown his way. When Algernon died, Charlie brought flowers, thus giving the story its heart-breaking title. Mrs. Hewitt and most of us had tears in our eyes that September afternoon as we sensed the powerful kinship of man, mouse, and tragedy.

"I'm like Algernon," I thought, wiping away my own tears in the Headway day room forty-some years after hearing the story. That's what we're all like here. We went through third grade to learn how to subtract and now we fumble at the simplest numbers. We went through high school and college and learned how to solve problems, and now simple subtraction was impossible. Algernon collapsed. So had I. Literature told the truth, and although it was a truth we would not choose of our own accord, it was somehow comforting to know I was not alone. The afternoon drew to its close. I left the day room and headed outside to find my ride back home. The cell phone rang. It was Connie.[9]

9 Wanting to thank Jan Hewitt fifty-some years after her reading, I sent her this chapter in September, 2009. Now teaching at Rice University, she remembered that afternoon with all its emotional clarity. "Unless I miss my guess", I wrote, "I bet you still read stories out loud with your classes." "We never know how our words and actions will affect others, even far in the future," she wrote back. "You have validated the influence of teaching and of meaningful literature. You will be astonished to learn that I [visited another Euclid teacher this past June], and she and I talked about my reading *Flowers for Algernon*, and how I cried at the ending. You are right about my continuing to read aloud."

"Larry," she said, "They got the results from the MRI. You need to go back in and see Dr. Gumm. They've given the results to him." It didn't occur to me that she didn't want to share them with me over the phone. Neither did I appreciate that she and David had talked about the best way to break the news. I was glad it would be David, not a neurologist. David was a healer, not a technician, and I had long since lost my trust in neurologists. I headed back to Headway, pushed the LL button once again and walked down the art-filled hallway to David's office.

"So, what's up?" I asked, eager to know. My words were clear, without a trace of aphasia. I was sure I'd had a somewhat major TIA, that was all. It would be a warning but not a lasting problem. My slowness at the arithmetic problems was probably just a matter of fatigue.

"Do you have the results?" I asked.

"Yes," he said. "It was a stroke."

"It was?"

"Yes. I'm sorry," mixing compassion and concern. "It was on the left side."

"Oh my," I said. "The left side?" Now I understood why the subtraction problem that I could have done a week earlier was suddenly a bridge too far. If the stroke hit a language center no wonder I could not find words. My case had just become more complicated. The precarious predictions that he and Kirby had foreseen, that I was far more fragile than I realized had proved to be true. The right side had its Antarctica. And now the left side had an ice flow of its own. It was small, showing an area of dead cells no larger than a small nut. Disability now had symmetry and I could not subtract 18 from 34.

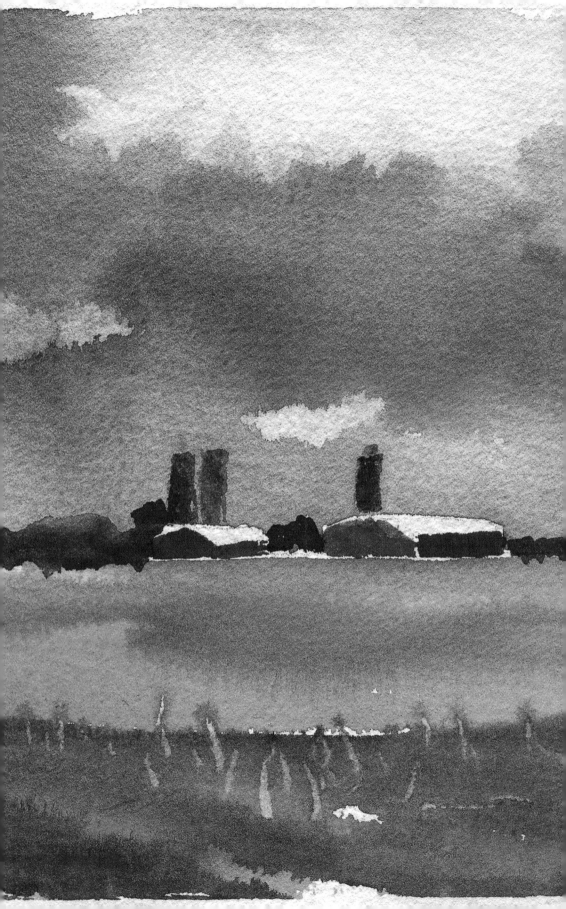

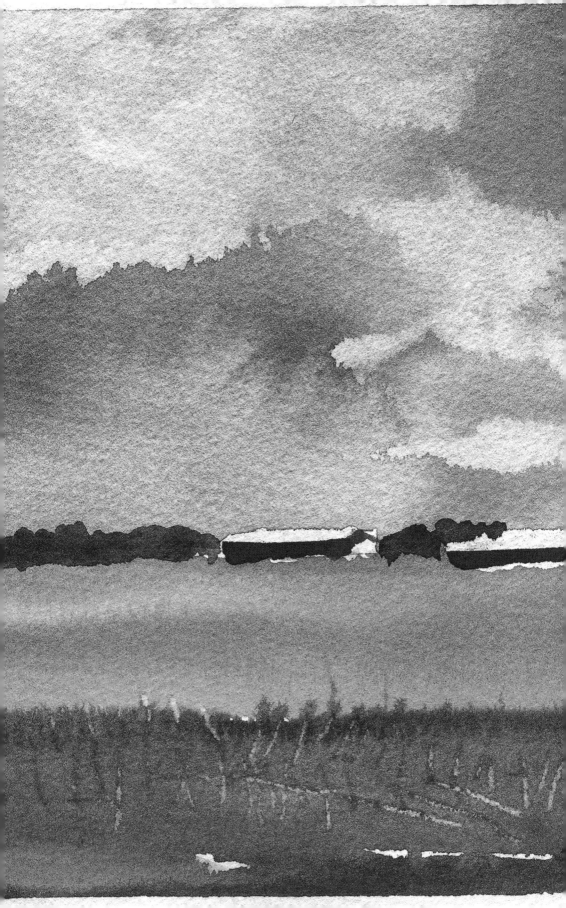

chapter fifteen
offloading

•••

Coherence has a memory.

I am perhaps ten years old and my father and I are in the aisle of the Rexall Drug store in Littleton, Colorado. We are there to purchase a spare glass syringe and a few steel needles to replace those we have been sharpening on the whetstone, another brown bottle of isopropyl alcohol to keep both needle and syringe sterile and a few vials of insulin. We are there to pick up the supplies of nothing less than life.

The pharmacist greets us by name as we make our way down the aisle to the chest-high counter where the pharmacy begins and the sundries end. There is a bit of easy conversation, perhaps about the weather, perhaps just a, "How have you been?" perhaps some take on the headlines of the day. "We'll take four bottles of insulin," says my dad. The pharmacist opens the door of the small refrigerator and reaches for the bottles of insulin. My dad pays for them, we give our thanks, and begin to walk down the aisle, wondering if we've forgotten anything, perhaps a box of cotton balls, marked with the word STERILE, or something my mother had asked him to pick up.

We leave the store knowing that once again life has been resupplied and chaos tamed. We never say, "Without this drug store, without those syringes, without the fresh supply of insulin it would all be over in a few days." There is no fear in these visits. Instead there is safety, balance and harmony. All is well, God is nigh.

Coherence has a memory. It is no surprise believers and nonbelievers both know about Eden. It is no surprise that the creation story brings order out of chaos, and that Adam and Eve find themselves in a place where all things can work to the good, where only the perception of scarcity can bring abundance to an end. Coherence has an enduring memory both in scripture and in our lives.

Half a century later the memories of Rexall Drug surround me when I walk into Cole Drug in Big Timber, Montana, approach the chest-high counter at the end of the aisle and ask Doug or Stormy for a bottle of insulin. We also talk for a while, noting the wind, the snow or the heat that threatens to ignite the air itself. They also reach into the small refrigerator for the small white boxes of genetically engineered insulin. I thank them, walk back down the aisle with its assortment of plastic syringes, and pay the bill at the front of the store. Once again all is well. Once again, order prevails, once again all things work on behalf of healing.

The memory of coherence makes connection a necessity. The pharmacists, my doctor who wrote the prescription, the insurance company that helps cover its hefty price, the church that called me and paid me as pastor, the Eli Lilly company that manufactures and delivers a new kind of insulin every decade or so, all work together to keep chaos at bay. We trust these connections, we rely on their healing presence, we guard them, protect them and come to expect them.

And, in each of our lives, there comes a day when they begin to crumble. Such a vulnerability is not entirely unexpected. The levees that protect New Orleans have their limits. The serpent's temptation was fierce enough to crack Eden's harmony and launch us on a life-long journey to mend a broken world.

History also tells the story of these epic struggles. Connie is Cherokee, and the shelves of books that line the walls of our small apartment tell the same story, over and over again. We talk one evening about this chapter. She reminds me of the Sand Creek massacre in November 1864 when Black Kettle had been told that if he just flew an American flag over his tepee both he and his people would always be protected. Indeed he had a medal he could show to any enemy that would ensure safe passage. But it made no difference when the soldiers attacked the mostly old men, women and children, killing more than 200. Black Kettle died holding the medal in his hands. The Cheyenne, the Cherokee, the Lakota, the Nez Pierce, the Palestinians, the Acadians were all offloaded to some other place when chaos assaulted coherence and sowed the seeds of anguish.

The prophet Amos spoke eloquently about the plight of those who sought safety of a flag, a Rexall Drug Store, shelter from a storm named Katrina, or treatment for brain injury at Walter Reed Hospital and found themselves abandoned:

> It is as if someone fled from a lion and was met by a bear;
> or went into a house and rested a hand against a wall
> and was bitten by a snake. (Amos 5:19)

We had the disability insurance offered through our denomination. Within days of the first stroke Connie made the requisite calls and received assurance that assistance would be provided. The glossy pamphlet describing benefits led us to give thanks that we had disability insurance. We would be okay. An initial check arrived to tide us over as medical bills escalated with an ever-increasing urgency. Connie sheltered me from the full force of the bills, fearing the stress might trigger another stroke. I floated incoherently with the expectation that all was well, that I would soon be back at work, that the insurance system would work. As so often happens in financially frail institutions, confusion began to present itself. The expected checks did not arrive, the form Connie needed to fill out to receive those checks was sent but then could not be located. A local attorney offered his services *pro bono* and arranged for a power of attorney form to be signed. With comprehension on the wane, and an inability to understand the situation we faced, to say nothing of my lack of judgment, Connie shouldered the full load of our financial affairs. She did so as her own condition became increasingly frail. For her, too, simple tasks required days of recovery, and travel became almost impossible.

The church helped out, with grace-filled generosity, taking up a special collection to help pay the medical bills.

John Schaeffer contacted a denominational emergency fund for ministers that had helped us before.

The few resources we had were sent away to pay down the escalating bills. We put our home up for sale.

We had been talking with the disability office of our denomination, grateful for the assistance and assurance of its presence. The brochures about disability insurance were reassuring, as glossy brochures often are. After an initial flurry of compassion a new tone and a new set of questions began to emerge. Were we facing short-term disability or would it be long-term disability? To our surprise it wasn't the denomination that wanted to know...it was a secular insurance company we had never heard of. The denomination responsible for the spiritual discernment of call had outsourced disability to a commercial insurance company. We were no longer in the province of faith. Economics would rule the day, and our needs, to say nothing of call or ministry, would have to play second fiddle. Would our disability be short-term or long-term? Were these expenses to be temporary? Or might they be long-term? The insurance company wanted to know.

Were the homes along the Gulf Coast destroyed as a result of wind? Or was it water? The insurance companies wanted to know. The plight of the family who lost a home was a secondary consideration. Costs came first. It was as though the pharmacist at Rexall Drug began to say, "How many times will you have to keep returning for insulin? How long will this disability last?" "A long time" would not be the right answer. To avoid its cost and complexity the denomination offloaded disability to an insurance company that in turn would do everything it could to offload us onto the shoulders of the government. The piercing question W.E.B. DuBois asked regarding race applied to us as well: "How does it feel to be a problem?"

There are few circumstances in life more alluring than short-term problems. We celebrate treatments that work, problems that can be fixed once and for all. In such cases we gather our resources, draw on the goodwill of friends and family, address the problem and return to the rhythms of life. There is something heroic about solving short-term problems. Together we sandbag the river, wait for the rain to stop falling and, before long, we find a short-term solution. And there are few circumstances in life more daunting than long-term problems that linger and linger. Cronus was the destructive Greek god of time who devoured each of his children as soon as they were born. When his wife, Rhea, realized what he was doing she intervened to save Zeus by wrapping a stone in swaddling clothes and telling Cronus it was Zeus. When we call a disease and the lack of finances "chronic" we enter this exceedingly difficult realm in which the intervention of loving friends is the only antidote to ruthless power. But Cronus swallowed many children, and the realm of chronic illness can be a fearful place in which we often find ourselves alone.

At first disability is the problem. Then long-term disability deepens the problem. And then we realize that we are the problem. In February, an anticipated check from the insurance company did not arrive. In March it did not arrive, but the second stroke did. Forms from people we did not know arrived, forms were sent to people we did not know. We complied and were told we had not complied. Confusion reigned and fear made its presence known. We were surrounded and confused by the "fog of war." Our concern was survival. The insurance company wanted to know how expensive that might be.

After the March stroke both Connie and Kirby knew that we had to leave town. The controlled situation essential to survival could not be found in Big Timber. They knew my mind would always be on the church, that a visit to the post office would always involve picking up the social mail as well as letters in the mailbox. They knew that the intersection of a pastor with parishioners is always full of meaning. How are you...really? I heard that...Let's talk. Meet you for coffee. Every store, every house, every church had its story just waiting for an added chapter. We had to find a neutral place. Connie looked for an apartment in Billings but came up empty. She finally found an apartment in Red Lodge, a tourist town at the base of the Beartooth Mountains that would allow us to bring Casey. It was a very small apartment, perhaps the equivalent of a FEMA trailer that would have to suffice for home. Each day brought relief that a third stroke had not struck. Each day brought another round of bills that without the expected checks we could not pay.

On the way to make arrangements for the small apartment Connie called the denomination's executive assigned to field the needs of clergy caught by crisis. The executive had an unenviable position. By and large clergy are a remarkably unhealthy group of people and when we encounter a serious health crisis we generally have few resources to face it down. The resources at the denomination's disposal were as limited as the resources of those making a worrisome emergency call. Neither could square what they would like to do with financial reality. Saying "yes" to every plea meant saying "no" to the next set of pleas. Scripture has a word for such an impasse. There were not enough fish and not enough loaves to feed the five thousand gathered on a Galilean hillside. But instead of breaking off from the crowd, Jesus and the disciples stayed with the crowd and blessed the few resources they had. Community, not scarcity, was the final word.

And so Connie made the call. If something had gone wrong perhaps it could be fixed. If there was something she had not done perhaps she would learn what it was. If there was a misunderstanding certainly it could be cleared up. Her call would set things right. Connie explained the situation and received a reprimand. If we had sensed before that we were the problem Cronus had framed, she now knew it for sure. She must have done something wrong and the last thing anyone needed was another problem.

One day, driving from Billings to Red Lodge, the enormity of the crisis hit full force. Fighting back the pain of her own disability that even years on the morphine pump could not take away, and the tears from the crisis at hand, Connie pulled off the road. A Highway Patrol officer noticed her collapsed on the steering wheel. He slowed down, turned around, and came back. He came over to the car, heard her sobs, and tapped at the window.

"Are you okay?" he gently asked.

"I'll be okay," she said. "Thank you."

"Take your time," he said. "Can I help at all?"

"No," she said.

"Take care," he said.

Tone tells the story. He was not angry. He did not order her off the road. He asked if she was okay knowing that something had been offloaded into her life that was too heavy a burden to carry alone. There is a story in the life of the prophet Elijah that continued to reveal itself to us over the years. In a time of great fear, Elijah expected to find God in the wind, but God was not in the wind. He expected to find God in the fire, but God was not in the fire. He expected to find God in the earthquake, but God was not in the earthquake. Instead, God spoke in a still small voice. Connie expected to find hope at the 911 desk but it was not found there. Instead God sent the gentle presence of a Highway Patrol officer who let her know she was not alone.

Our oldest son returned home from Los Angeles to pack up our belongings and put them into storage. At one point I said, "Why? We're not moving. We can just rent the house as it is, we'll be home soon. We're not moving." Once again anosognosia tried to create its own reality. Tim began the offloading of our possessions into a metal storage unit on the edge of town. He then loaded a U-Haul with remnants of our possessions and with the help of parishioners, moved us to Red Lodge, Montana.

New letters began to arrive each with an IF-THEN construction. IF we were to be on long-term disability THEN Medicare would have to pick up most of the tab. The letters made it clear that no long-term claims would be accepted without qualifying for Social Security. Another letter arrived, this one requesting more forms. Why had we not returned the forms? Why had we not answered the phone? Why weren't we Johnny-on-the-spot? Connie sorted through the notebook of correspondence she had carefully kept. She couldn't find the required forms. Had they been lost when mail had to be forwarded from 59011 to 59068? Had the insurance company tried to call us when I was at rehab and she was napping to fend off the pain and the hurricane of stress she carried? The computer-generated letter insisted that IF the forms were not received in three days THEN all benefits would stop. Rightly or wrongly we understood all benefits referred to both a monthly check and our health insurance. I had to somehow get on Medicare, without which all would come to a halt. It dawned on us that taking care of us was not in their economic interest. Our survival cost them money they would perhaps prefer not to pay.

Connie placed yet another call, this time to the insurance company.

"We haven't received the forms you're asking for," she said.

"We must have them in three days."

"But there are no forms."

"Yes there are. We sent them. You have three days to comply."

I was at Headway where the problems involved subtraction and addition.

How do you subtract 38 from 64? Meanwhile Connie faced the subtractions and additions upon which our lives depended. If something could not be done Rexall Drug would disappear. She drove from the hospital, spotted an attorney's office and walked in.

"I need help," she said.

"May I ask your name?" the secretary said.

"Connie Pray," Connie said. "And I need help. My husband's at the hospital and I don't know where to turn."

The secretary buzzed an attorney to let him know a woman had just walked in who needed some emergency help with an insurance claim. Chances were better than even that his reply would be, "So?" But that is not what he said.

"Show her in," he said. Connie walked into his office, her bag full of correspondence. She shared the string of IF-THENs and the threat of the three-day window. The attorney was aghast.

"This is the work of the church?"

"Yes. No. It's been outsourced. It's an insurance company."

"This is the response of the government?" a nation asked after Katrina.

"This is the care our soldiers receive?" a nation asked as TBI soldiers at Walter Reed found their aftercare denied and their return to life neglected.

Then the attorney did what attorneys do. He reached for a phone and called the company. "I have a client," he said, "who has been told to do the impossible. I've looked over her records and believe there is a problem on your end. I'm quite sure this is not what you intend. I would like for you to fax the forms to my office this afternoon." Within minutes the office phone began to ring and the fax began to spew forth eleven pages of forms.

Scripture assures us that there are times the Spirit intercedes with sighs too deep for words. In the month of March, when tired banks of dirty snow lined the roads, when Connie carried the cargo of our life on her shoulders without my full recognition of how heavy a load it was, when tears carried unspoken prayers, a Highway Patrol officer whose name we did not know, and an attorney whose presence we could not have expected, appeared. The capacity for prayer had disappeared but the abiding presence of the Spirit had not. Vestiges of Rexall

Drug remained. Coherence always has unexpected helpers. Life's healing river cannot be fully dammed.

Would it be long-term or short-term? Social Security read the reports from Kirby and Headway, examined the MRI and the CAT scans and added me to their roles within just a few weeks. The long-term diagnosis took its first few steps in Red Lodge, Montana.

chapter sixteen
reconstruction 101

• • •

I knew it was a keeper.

"Love the pitcher less, the water more," read the Sufi maxim. The water could be God and the pitcher our interpretations of God. Both mattered. If one tended only to the water and ignored the pitcher, how could the water be shared? But if one tended only to the pitcher, and became consumed by whether it was made of tin or of glass, the pitcher might take the place of the water it was created to carry.

Either way the sentence makes sense, and either way I had work to do. It was not enough to wake up each day, see if I could make sense of a puzzle, walk the dog, bake a loaf of bread and fetch the ingredients for supper, as Connie no longer had the capacity to do either, and wait for the next day at Headway. All of that was to the good, but not enough. The still empty spiritual pitcher needed to find its water. The confidence I once had in my intellect needed a serious workout. Although my IQ had taken a hit, perhaps it could be regained if I did some homework. Headway had given me math problems as part of rehab. What if I tackled some spiritual problems?

On my bookshelf was a pale yellow book that somehow survived our move from Big Timber to Red Lodge. Many of its pages were earmarked, and had notes or questions written in the margins. *Early Christian Doctrines*, by J. N. D. Kelley[10] is one of the premiere church history texts. I first read it not because I wanted to, but because it was part of the required reading at seminary. At the time it seemed like a remote academic pursuit. Over time, I learned that at its core church history reflects what people and cultures do with the idea of "God." Its

---

10 *Early Christian Doctrines*, revised edition, J.N.D. Kelley, Harper Collins, New York, 1978

studies of the pitcher could be violent, heartbreaking, inspiring, and eloquent over the course of time. The first sentence of the book set the stage for my study.

"The object of this book is to sketch the development of the principal Christian doctrines from the close of the first century to the middle of the fifth," Kelly wrote in the first sentence of his book.

"That's perfect," I said to myself. "My object is to trace the development of Christian doctrine in my life from the days it began to disappear to the spring of 2004." The study required careful reading, note taking, and many second reads. I put aside the 20-minute restriction on reading, did what I could and when fatigue took its toll, tried to get some exercise, often thinking about what I'd just read and wondering what to do with it.

Some of the text was heavy sledding, and read a bit like medical notes. "Aristobulus had used [allegorical exegesis] to explain away the cruder anthropomorphisms of the Pentateuch. Philo takes it up enthusiastically, and contends that, of the various attitudes possible to the Mosaic Law, much the most satisfactory is to observe its prescriptions punctiliously while at the same time striving with the aid of allegory to grasp their deeper purport." Hmmm... interesting. But bit by bit the pieces of the Christological puzzle began to fall into place. For Philo, God's pure being was so absolutely transcendent it was "without quality." The thought resonated with the first hymn in the United Church of Christ hymnal, *Immortal, Invisible, God Only Wise*, whose first verse asserts God's presence "in light inaccessible hid from our eyes."

I liked that, but the invisible asked for some attention. In each chapter, Kelly presented a new thinker. To Irenaeus, a bishop in southern France (then known as Gaul) Jesus and the Spirit were both vehicles of divine revelation. After all, he reasoned, if God is spiritual, God must have a spirit too, so while there is one God this one God has different aspects of which Jesus is one. But over in Byzantium, a theologian, Theodotus, insisted Jesus was a human being just like everyone else who then received an indwelling of the spirit that signaled his adoption. Not so, said other thinkers who noted that single objects have many aspects. After all, light that comes from the sun is not the same thing as the sun.

And so it went. Each chapter also presented an argument that somehow asked me to choose sides. Rigorous as the study was, it did not fill my spirit. Then two words that appeared on Kelley's densely written pages, triggered a memory. The history professor had taken a piece of chalk and written a single Greek word:

Homousias.

It means, he said, "of the same substance." There were those who believed, and believe, that Jesus is of the very same substance as God.

Then he wrote a second word: *Homoiusias.* It meant, "Of the same essence." The adding of a single "i" brought about a vast change.

Head Ed was just a few days away, and I knew I had something to share with David and the group. It was his class, but I could hardly wait to bring 2,000 years of church history to the fore.

I took a thick felt marker and wrote the words *homousias* and *homoiusias* on the board behind David. By then we knew each other's stories, and sensed the progress we were or were not making. Would our new life be *homousian* or *homoiusian*? We had all sustained too much damage to build a new life out of the same substance. But had our essence changed as well? The theological reflections weren't theological at all. Instead they lay at the heart of rehabilitation.

"I believe that although we have changed, we still have the same essence we once did," I said. "I know we have changed. I know we can scarcely recognize ourselves. But these changes have not eroded our essence. Down deep we are who we were. Even if this is not true physically, it is certainly true spiritually. This gives me hope and perhaps it can give us hope as well."

They got it. We who had trouble thinking, whose IQs had diminished, understood immediately the deep dialogue between substance and essence. Two thousand years of church history fought over it. We lived it.

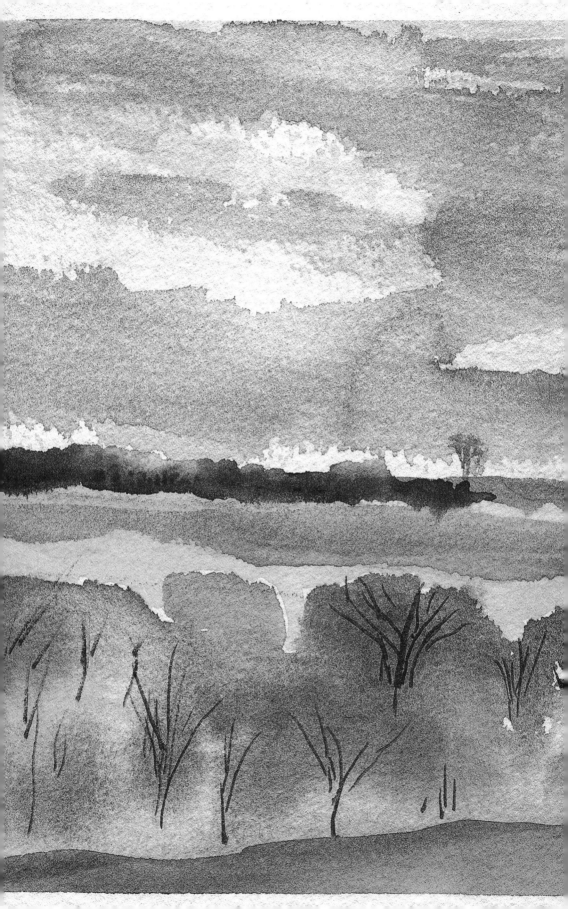

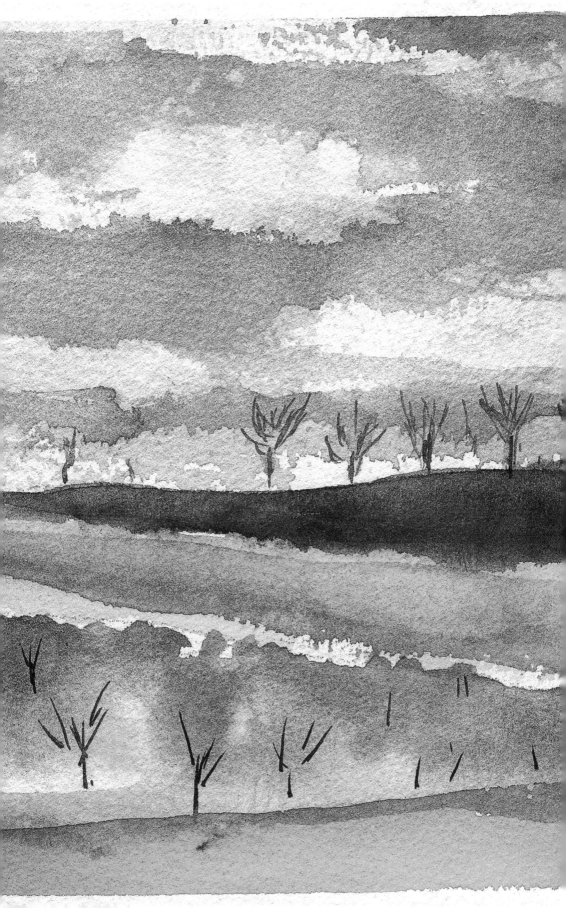

chapter seventeen
the drive

...

Months had passed since my seizure. I assumed that the prospect of another seizure was the only reason I could not drive. The risk was understandable and the well-travelled road from Billings to Red Lodge was well known for its many accidents. Souvenir shops sold sweatshirts emblazoned with the words *I survived Highway 210*. Every few miles there was yet another set of small white crosses marking the site of a fatal accident. Sometimes a skier headed for the mountains hit a patch of ice; once an inebriated motorcycle rider collided with a cow. But I wanted to drive.

When I first asked about it, the occupational therapists said, "Not until the doctors give the go ahead." Headway would let us know when that day arrived. One day, to my surprise, Catherine said it was time for a test drive. The rehabilitation unit had a car designed for just such an event. Like cars outfitted for drivers' education classes, it had two sets of brakes. It was not a Porsche or a Ferrari, did not have stick shift. It was a remarkably level-headed vehicle. Forty years of driving had resulted in only one ticket (which certainly wasn't my fault) and one accident (I looked left; I looked right; I looked straight ahead; and then I pulled out and hit the oncoming car). She unlocked the driver's door, I got in and took care to quickly fasten the seatbelt as if to say, "See! You thought I might forget but I didn't!" I would pass the driving test with flying colors. I turned the key, heard the engine kick in, carefully backed up, and headed for the exit.

"Turn left here," Catherine said after we left the garage.

I turned left.

"Now let's go straight into the neighborhood across the street."

"Okay," I said. I waited for the green light and gingerly headed across the street. Like a 16-year old taking his driving test, I was ever so cautious. The neighborhood was somewhat familiar to me as 35 years earlier I had rented a tiny apartment there when I first came to Montana to work as a cub reporter for the *Billings Gazette.* Covering fires and the police beat were parts of my responsibility. It never ceased to amaze me that Billings had two fire departments—one public, and one private. People outside of the city limits subscribed to the private fire company. It was understood the company would only put out customer's fires. If the house next door burned down and wasn't on the company's list, that was just too bad.

"I didn't know that," said Catherine.

"Yes," I said, realizing I shouldn't have been talking and driving at the same time.

"Now turn here."

"Okay."

"Let's go up to the light." We went up to the light. Every correct turn, every proper waiting for other cars to pass, every anticipated action felt like a victory. After about 15 minutes we headed back to Headway. I drove into the garage, returned to the parking spot designated for the car, carefully slid into the space, set the brake, turned off the engine and handed Catherine the keys. We walked into the day room.

Adrenalin is a remarkable drug. There are times that we feel its surge as it strengthens us and turns random thoughts into streams of pure emotion. But there are other times when we are scarcely aware of its presence until it seemingly evaporates and leaves us utterly spent. As soon as I walked through the doors of the day room I felt my entire body collapse. There is, in the day room, a very soft recliner. I rarely sat in it, preferring the hard chairs that would help focus my attention. Hard chars felt industrious. Easy chairs lived up to their brand name: Lay-Z-Boy. I looked at the chair; cast aside my normal inclinations and sat down on its soft cushions. I was utterly, unexpectedly and completely exhausted. The world of expectation that said, "I can do this, I will pass this, I will be able to drive again just as I did before" had no chance.

I thought that my seizures were the impediment to driving. Now I realized the seizures were the least of my worries. I did not have the strength to endure a 15 minute drive. Once upon a time all the cells in my brain noticed oncoming traffic, computed what I should do about it, paid attention to the colors, the sounds, the conversation, the light, the gas tank, the speedometer, how much time had passed for the allotted drive, what I might say when I arrived at the store, where my checkbook was, how much money it did or didn't have, what I was supposed to buy, what I wanted to buy, who was on the street, when the sun would go down and what kind of weather the clouds promised. All of these computations happened automatically.

For years I had wondered why driving is tiring. Now I knew.

Noting my collapse, and checking again with the doctors, Catherine told me that it was still too dangerous for me to drive. Curiously enough, if I had felt fatigue coming on as I drove it would be safer. If that happened I would simply pull over, find a quiet place and sleep for a spell. But part of the mystery of brain injury is that it takes time for the full nature of fatigue to reveal itself.

I asked David about the furtive nature of fatigue.

"The ebb in strength and energy that all people experience is analogous to running out of gas in a car," he said. "There may be no warning before the fuel is gone and the vehicle can't go on. The difference between the non brain-injured and the brain-injured is that the brain-injured person has a much smaller tank now. They don't perceive it that way, though. They assume, just as you did, that the tank is the same size it always was. The task for the injured person is to acknowledge that the tank is smaller and plan accordingly. You have to adapt. This, of course, is difficult when anosognosia blocks the perception of disability in the first place."

He then gave a scientific explanation.

"Energy utilization is a series of biological events that involve mitochondria, which make up the cell's power plant. There are a number of possible sources of energy/fatigue problems following brain injury that include changes in endocrine/pituitary and hypothalamus functioning; cell membrane changes; mitochondrial changes; changes in the sodium and potassium levels, to name a few possibilities.

In your case the situation is made far more complex by diabetes.

"Overall the fatigue experienced is most likely a response to the amount of energy expended. However energy is expended by the brain in unpredictable ways. So a happy event like a wedding or family gathering may require more energy than walking five miles or working out every day as you've continued to do. Cognitively complex situations may demand more energy than physically demanding ones. The reorganization of the brain as part of the healing process is a slow, steady event, which does undoubtedly contribute to the overall fatigue, but is probably not the main cause of the acute fatigue that sets a person back for several days."

There was nothing to do but wait, and learn again what could and could not be done. A month or so later, in the late spring of 2004, I received permission to drive.

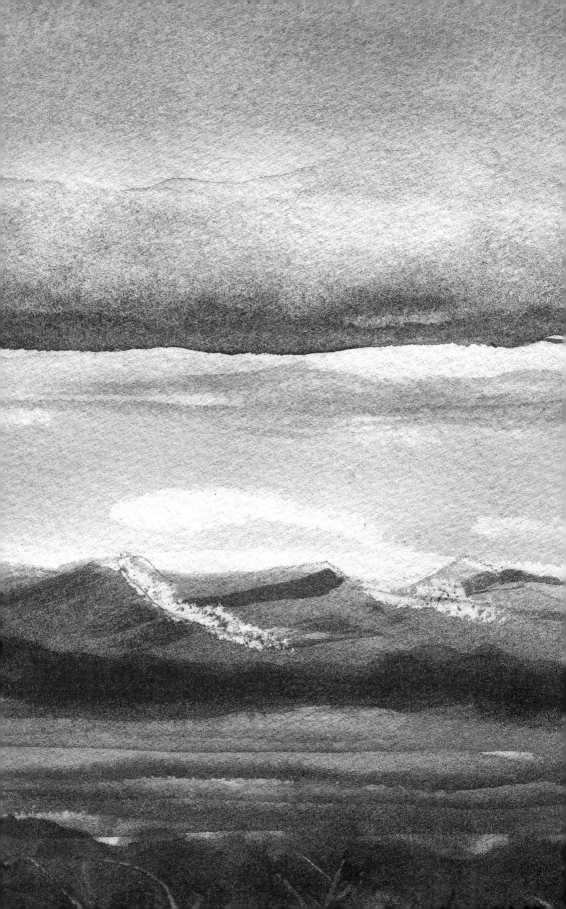

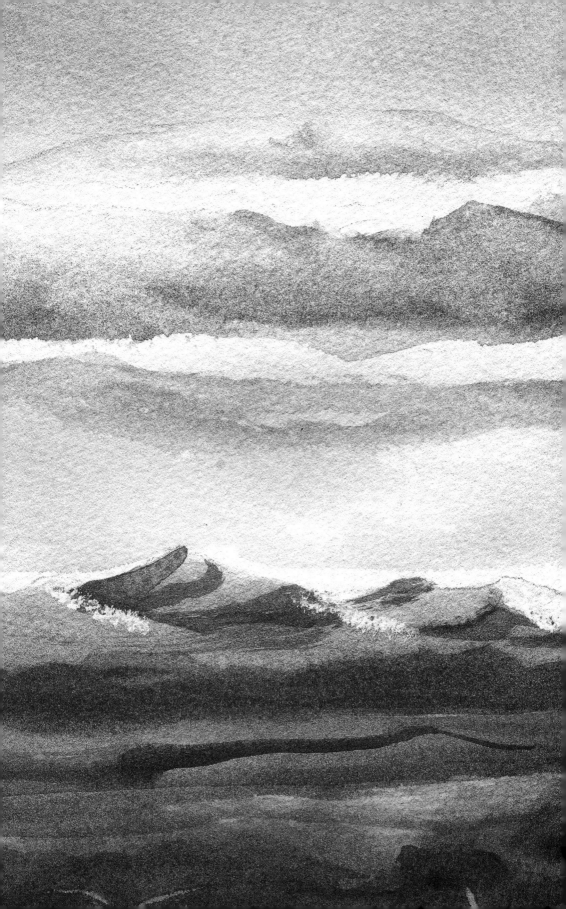

chapter eighteen
communion

• • •

The church in Red Lodge greeted us with open arms and a depth of hospitality. Its pastor, David Munson, was a perfect match for the vitality of a congregation that blended pastoral care and prophetic witness with conviction and serenity. We shared many walks piecing together the rehab and what the future held. When I spoke of being thrown overboard, my disillusioned words were laden with more than a tinge of anger. Just as Kirby had said on the first day of the stroke, "The man before me was not Larry Pray," I sensed that David was not quite sure I was the same person he had once known. I kept getting "stuck" on outrage, knowing that was the last thing I wanted to do. Getting "stuck" is one symptom of brain damage. Besides, the "victory" I expected from Headway was ever so elusive, and the second stroke had indeed set me back. In short, hope was in short supply.

One of the elders had said, "Larry, we want to be your church." I wanted to be part of their church as well, and wondered how to fit into its cornucopia of activities when I had been told to stay in controlled settings. There was not one part of the Red Lodge liturgy that was too much. But when put together, it was more than I could handle. All those wonderful kids, all those announcements, hymns I knew but still couldn't sing, a well-delivered and thoughtful sermon, passing the offering--it drained me. When I attended a class or two, I stumbled a bit on what my role was, much as I had on the day I wasn't sure just what I was doing at a funeral, and what to say to the newly-engaged couple. I just couldn't make it work, and my pitcher remained empty. One Sunday, as strength slipped away, I quietly left the service before it ended to gather myself and begin a slow walk home. Knowing that few things are as disconcerting to a pastor than watching a parishioner, especially if he or she is a pastor, leave the middle of a service, I wrote David a note and slid it under his door the next day.

David,

I am so sorry I had to leave the service yesterday. It had nothing to do with your sermon, or anything you said, or anything you did. I just found that I couldn't keep up with all that was happening, and I could feel the life running out of me. I needed to go home. It is what the doctors said would happen if I wasn't in a controlled environment. I am so sorry. Everyone has been so kind and we appreciate your presence. Blessings to you.

Larry

The sacraments of life and worship would have to be found in other ways, in other places. It was, of course nothing new. There was a time in ancient Israel when worship had to take place in Jerusalem. Worship outside of the temple was considered to be a step away from the presence of God. But then the Babylonians invaded, destroyed the temple, and sent the survivors into exile. Suddenly the Israelites had to pray in new ways, understand God in new ways, and walk with God in new ways. The old ways, understandings and even places no longer held life. Some new listening had to happen. Before the strokes I had shared with the Big Timber congregation a Quaker hymn whose words and melody we took to heart. Though I could no longer sing, their serene message stayed with me as I wondered how to find the stride of worship once again. The hymn's title could not have been more fitting:

Teach Me to Stop and Listen[11]

Teach me to stop and listen
teach me to center down,
teach me the use of silence,
teach me where peace is found.

Teach me to hear your calling
teach me to search your words

---

11 *Teach Me to Stop and Listen*, by Ken Medema, four in Worship in Song, A Friends Hymnal, a publication of Friends General Conference, 1996, Philadelphia, Pennsylvania, p. 137.

Teach me to hear in silence
Things I have never heard.

Teach me to be collected
teach me to be in tune.
Teach me to be directed,
Silence will end so soon.

Then when it's time for moving
Grant it that I may bring
To every day and moment,
Peace from a silent spring.

For some reason I had a rule in Red Lodge, one that is still in place. I would never drive within town. If we needed groceries, I would walk to the store. When we needed to visit the pharmacy, same thing. Each walk downtown led me by the church and its square red brick steeple. Steeples were designed to serve a purpose. They rise higher than the buildings around them, saying to all who see them, "Look up here! Look up." They embody the ancient litany, "Lift up your hearts." "We lift our hearts to God," the people respond. Just seeing the steeple gave a measure of hope. I decided to try worship again.

One Sunday, before the benediction, I quietly headed for the door hoping to politely avoid the confusing bevy of greetings and side conversations that a good worship service and a healthy congregation always inspire. Just outside the church door a flock of cedar waxwings had gathered in a sumac tree that still contained clusters of its bright scarlet berries. The tree virtually shimmered with their sunlit wings. There might have been twenty or more of them perched on the branches of that small tree. To my astonishment, they had not taken wing when the door opened. Instead, they stayed in the tree, moving a little this way, then a little that way. The tree quietly shuddered with their movements that were utterly without fear.

A moment later that door opened again as a few more people came out of church into the morning's sunlight. Still the waxwings held their place. Two or three of us, then four or five of us quietly marveled at their fearless presence. I stepped forward. Still they stayed. I stepped forward again. They were not startled. I waited. And then, as if by some silent command they all spread their wings and flew into the sky. We heard and felt the flutter of their beautiful wings as they took flight. I sensed with inner certainty they were a living benediction that spoke in a language that touched my heart, mind, and soul and at long last lifted prayers I could not send into the heavens. As I write these words four years later, I still see them in the morning light, feel the flutter of their wings. That morning, when I saw that tree, those cedar waxwings were what I saw with my heart, mind and soul.

They were the stuff of vision that sparks a sacred conversation.

"What do you see?" God once asked the prophet Amos.

"A basket of fruit," Amos, replied. Amos was not told what he should see. He was simply asked to say what he saw. Then the divine conversation could began.

As it was with Amos so it was with Jeremiah.

"What do you see, Jeremiah?" God asked.

"I see the branch of an almond tree," said Jeremiah.

"You have seen well," said God. And then the conversation began.

It always struck me how utterly honest the prophets were when they said what they saw, without yet realizing where the vision would lead. Who would have thought an almond branch would launch the book of Jeremiah? It seemed like such a small thing. But it began a divine conversation. When the cedar waxwings took flight I saw and felt the return of prayer, as burdened words were effortlessly lifted into the sky. A new language, in a new place, had found its way.

And so it was with communion.

Her name was Lindy and she had fallen while rock climbing in Utah. The fall crushed part of her spine and sent her into a coma. With great effort she could speak, with equally great effort she could take a few steps. The extent of her injuries could only be matched by the courage she summoned to recover. Her parents and boyfriend, who was with her on the day she fell, surrounded her with love. She had an entire community pulling for her. Rehabilitation understands that healing is not a lonely experience. Although there is a place in medical care for HIPPA regulations that seal and shield a patient's medical history and diagnoses from the communities that might care for them, rehabilitation is facilitated when patients freely share their stories and care for each other. And so we knew something of Lindy's story and she knew something of ours.

It was about three in the afternoon in late April, as the day's therapies drew to their close. She had spent the afternoon baking bread with one of the occupational therapists. Its fragrant smell drifted out of the kitchen and into in the day room. We heard the door open, and looked over to see her, her boyfriend and therapist walk into the day room. Rarely are effort, courage and commitment so completely devoid of comparison as they are in rehabilitation. Nobody would ever say, "But you should be walking faster," or "How could you have missed that problem?" Faster does not always mean better, and more is not necessarily a blessing. Many times David emphasized that those who recover best from TBI or strokes are those who accept their new lot in life and live with it instead of trying to defeat it each and every day. It takes the proverbial "Type A" longer to heal than "Type B." It was a word of wisdom I did not want to hear as we and the church awaited to see what would happen when rehab came to an end. Although insurance companies insist on quick, progressive, and verifiable results, such an orientation is not always in keeping with healing.

As they walked into the room we greeted them and noticed the loaf the therapist carried and a small piece of bread in Lindy's hand.

I walked over to savor the loaf and to congratulate her.

"Larry," she said, drawing the word out with concentrated effort. It was the first time I had heard her say my name as her days of rehabilitation and mine rarely coincided. "Yes," I said. And then, forming each word with exquisite care, she handed me the piece of bread and said,

"This is for you."

She had used the words of communion. "This is the body of Christ," we say when sharing the bread during communion, "broken for you." The depth of kinship, patient to patient, the giving of gifts, the price of her gift all spoke of sacrament.

"Thank you," I said, thinking, "this is the bread of life."

The waxwings spoke of benediction and prayer; Lindy's words spoke of palpable sacrament. The Spirit had once again found a way to speak an unforgettable word of life.

"Come on over," Nicole, the occupational therapist, said, "let's play a game." She lifted a game called Cranium from its shelf and laid it out on the small table. There was a delicious irony in having brain-injured patients play a game called Cranium. Lindy took a seat, so did David, so did another patient or two, and so did Nicole. I had no idea how to play the game, but somehow there had to be a way to reach the winner's circle in middle of the board. Unlike the dice in most games Cranium's dice were octagons instead of squares, which is to say they threw me completely. It wasn't perfectly obvious which of the dice's eight numbers should hold sway after it was thrown. Along the way there was plenty to interpret: cards, colors, dice, and each other's position on the board.

Playing a new game with brain-injured patients is a highly recommended and unforgettable experience. None of us could quite remember whose turn it was, what we were supposed to do if the dice said "three" or "six" or "eight." David and Nicole knew, of course, and they gently guided the rest of us through the steps. I am used to being a leader. When communion is served I break the bread; when I enter a room I can't help but bend the discussion. If there is something to be done I will do it. But in this game I couldn't have been in charge if I wanted to; neither could the other patient, and neither could Lindy. And so we all took instruction, forgot instruction, and wrapped it all in laughter and gentle teasing.

David has a vivid memory of the sacramental afternoon.

"The game had multi-sided dice that showed a different number on each side. You were supposed to read the top number. You would say, 'Okay, I got it,' but then when it was your turn to throw the dice you would see all those numbers and just couldn't decide which one you were to use. You were just completely flummoxed. Getting the right one, and even knowing which one was on top required spatial reasoning and that is something you lost. You would say, 'Well, which number is it?' We'd say, "It's the top number." You would say 'okay,' but then you would read one of the others. I remember thinking it was a classic example of impaired visual spatial reasoning. You saw the numbers but could not decide which one applied to the game. I looked over to Nicole and she looked over at me because we both realized it showed the nature of your injury. You just couldn't process the numbers, absorb the various sequences of the game, or understand its rules."

David's memory was exactly right. I was indeed flummoxed. I couldn't figure it out. But the recollection of deficit is not my primary memory of that afternoon. I remember the laughter, the fellowship, the memory of a good time as three brain-injured patients played the indecipherable game known as Cranium.

Communion is a piece of bread and a cup of wine.

It is also a broken but beautiful fellowship. In the course of the afternoon there were no shoulds, no worries, no hidden obligations. There was an unexpected gift, carefully chosen words, and the pure pleasure of each other's company. I realized the joy of not being in charge. Our broken lives allowed life to speak in a communion of such utter simplicity it could only come from God.

It was communion separated from accomplishment.

It was the unexpected return of the sacred.

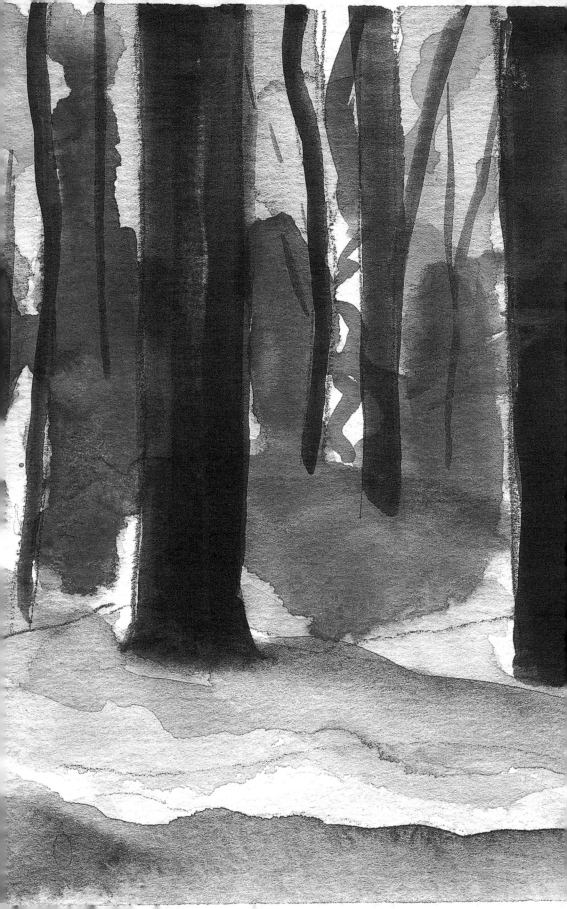

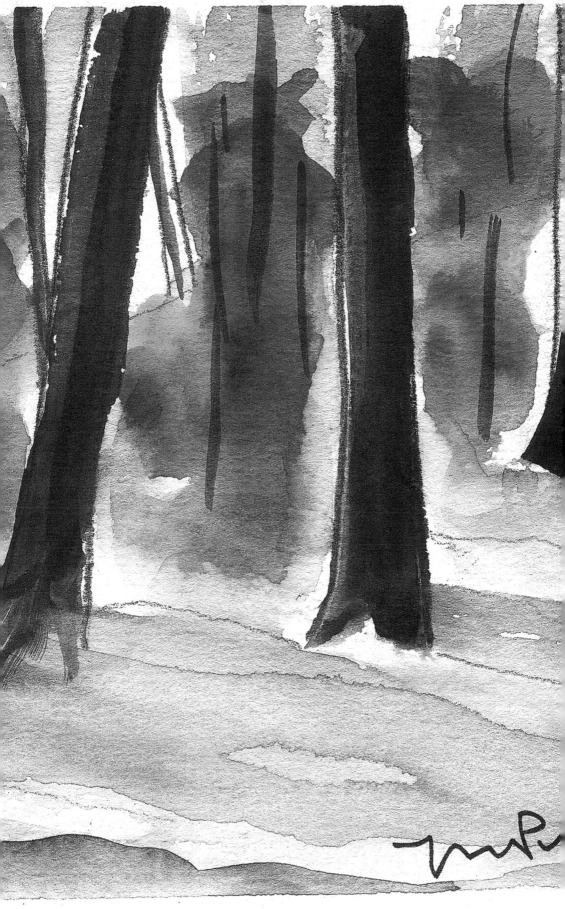

chapter nineteen
group

•••

By May, 2004, insurance had almost run its course. There were only so many days of rehabilitation they would cover. My voice had returned to its normal state. Sometimes I still mispronounced a word or two but inflection, though not rhythm and singing, had returned. Finally, almost six months after the first stroke I could recognize the person living in my skin. Wanting to bid a meaningful farewell to the therapists I wrote a poem for each one of them.

For Mary

> We first met you
> like Antarctic ice shelves
> that lost their home continent.
> One day, when no one saw it coming,
> they separated from the whole.
> Gently, you remind us
> that the ice in our minds
> is water, fresh water,
> that's been there since the beginning of time.
> "This is a great disconnect," you say.
> "But drink. You are fresh water in a salty sea."
> We let the currents go where they may.

In the letting go Connie wanted to find a way to keep rehabilitation alive and talked with David Gumm about the possibility of our starting a support group as part of the Headway curriculum. She knew it would be a form of ministry, that it would keep me in touch with Headway, and, most of all, that it was needed. The depth of fellowship that had grown among us as patients needed a formal and regular place in the Headway program. What had been serendipitous now deserved an ordered place and time. David, with his uncanny understanding of brain injury, and his grasp of healing as a process instead of a procedure, readily agreed with her. He would sit in on each session, but the floor would belong to the patients. I would be the facilitator. He had noticed that when I led a group there tended to be a depth of sharing. There was no explaining to be done. We were brain damaged, but we "got it." Our first gathering would be on my "graduation day."

Headway recognized the step from rehab to the "real world" called for and deserved careful attention. The files of puzzles we had tried to solve were handed back to us for safe keeping. On graduation day, someone ordered tacos, drinks, and all kinds of snacks. It was a heart-felt transition. All that could be done had been done. Life would now have to take care of itself. The AFLAC insurance agent could not return to his job. Neither could I. The future was uncertain at best. But we headed into it with a measure of thanksgiving for the progress that had been made by each patient and for the loving care we had received from each of the therapists. We decided this graduation day would be a picnic, that we would invite all of that year's Headway patients, their husbands or wives or lovers, their children, their cousins, all the staff, and the secretaries who worked behind the scenes, and anyone else that wanted to attend. And attend they did. After lunch I met with the stroke or brain injured patients and Connie met with their family members to sort through the experience of living with a changed person. In each gathering there was the sweet mixture of laughter and tears, of story and observation, of hope and the absence of hope. We laughed with Jackie who turned brain injury into an advantage by telling her husband she couldn't remember if he had kissed her goodnight or not and so she had no choice but to wake him up several times and receive a new round of kisses. We ached with Clela who had to organize her entire life according to the amount of energy she had. We joked that when we enter cafes and see someone sitting at a back table away from the din and commotion, he or she is probably a stroke or TBI survivor as that is exactly what we do.

Everyone in the group knew I was once a pastor but I was careful to share and elicit experience rather than belief. Whereas belief is narrow, always asking if one agrees or disagrees, experience is wide and carries with it the implicit trust of authenticity. In the course of our exchanges I asked if their injuries had changed their understanding of God, and if so, how? What they shared was simple, sometimes poignant, but their stories shared no predictable pattern. For some faith was the only certainty left in their lives. For others there was a sense that they needed to "do something" about the sacred part of their lives. We weren't sure just what form it took but there had to be something, somewhere, whether we could express it or not.

As it so often did, music sang what we could not say. The hymn *Over My Head*,[12] framed the search.

> *Over my head, I hear music in the air,*
> *over my head, I hear music in the air,*
> *over my head, I hear music in the air,*
> *I say, "There must be a God somewhere."*
>
> *Over my head, I hear trouble in the air,*
> *over my head, I hear trouble in the air*
> *over my head, I hear trouble in the air.*
> *I say, "There must be a God somewhere."*

Having the go-ahead to lead group, I drove from Red Lodge to Billings each Friday to meet with the Headway patients. One day, I decided to share the legend of St. George. For years I had been fascinated by a Russian icon showing a slender and slight St. George on a great stallion that crossed the iconic fields with astonishing power. In one hand he held reins as thin as string. Surely it would be impossible to control such a steed with such slender reins. And yet somehow, he kept his balance aboard the horse that had no intention of stopping. At the bottom of the icon, and off to one side, there was a dark cave from which a dragon emerged. We all knew exactly what the cave was: it was the lair of blood clots, of drunken drivers, of a surgery gone awry, of IED's, of the line drive from which there was no defense, the baseball bat used in a fight, the truck that drove

---

12 *Over My Head*, African-American traditional, New Century Hymnal, Pilgrim Press, 1995, Cleveland, Ohio.

too close to the horses alongside the road, the skull that leaked, or insurance companies that regretted what our lives cost them. We knew this cave like the back of our hand, and we knew the name of the dragon that did its best to end our ride.

In his other hand, St. George held a lance, not a sword. And therein lay the message.

"You will never see St. George holding the head of that dragon," I said to the group. "Killing the dragon isn't the goal. The goal is to simply pin him. We cannot "kill" our strokes or our injuries. We can't stop time. We can't go back. But we can pin the dragon that wants to—but hasn't been able to—throw us."

"I couldn't believe it when you said that," Steve said to me the next week. "All of a sudden I understood what I needed to do. It became clear. I had been trying to kill the dragon when all I needed to do was to pin him."

Group was, as Connie knew it would be, a blessing beyond words. Despite the 180 mile round-trip drive, and the cost of gas we could ill afford, it gave me "something to do," a way to lend a helping hand and a way to continue my own rehabilitation. In a sense it became my "church," its members my parishioners and, when I was out of gas they became my counselors. I saw, and was awed by, marriages that not only survived but grew despite the circumstances. I saw other patients graduate, and was thrilled when a month or two later they would drop by for "group," which had become a regular part of Headway.

Each week I stopped by the flower shop before leaving town and heading for Headway. Its owner, Phyllis, had heard about the group with a special interest. "I had an automobile accident 25 years ago," she shared. "I know how hard it is to come back, how long it takes to get back to life. When I went through it there was no such thing as group. So I want you to take these. It is the least I can do. So these are for the group." At the beginning of each session I placed the flowers on the small table that centered our circle. At the end of each session we chose who should receive the flowers. It wasn't a competition, it wasn't an evaluation. But with remarkable clarity the group seemed to sense exactly who would find the beautiful roses most beautiful.

Once they went to Carmen, who not only nearly lost her life but the lives of her horses as well when a truck collided with her and her horse trailer. Once they went to the family of the teenage pitcher who had been hit by a line drive and survived its resulting coma. Once they went to the woman who had no idea who her husband was when she awoke. Once they went to Dave; once to Lindsey; once to Peggy; once to David Gumm; once to Mandy; once to Jackie; once to Rita; once to…Each time the gift touched our soul.

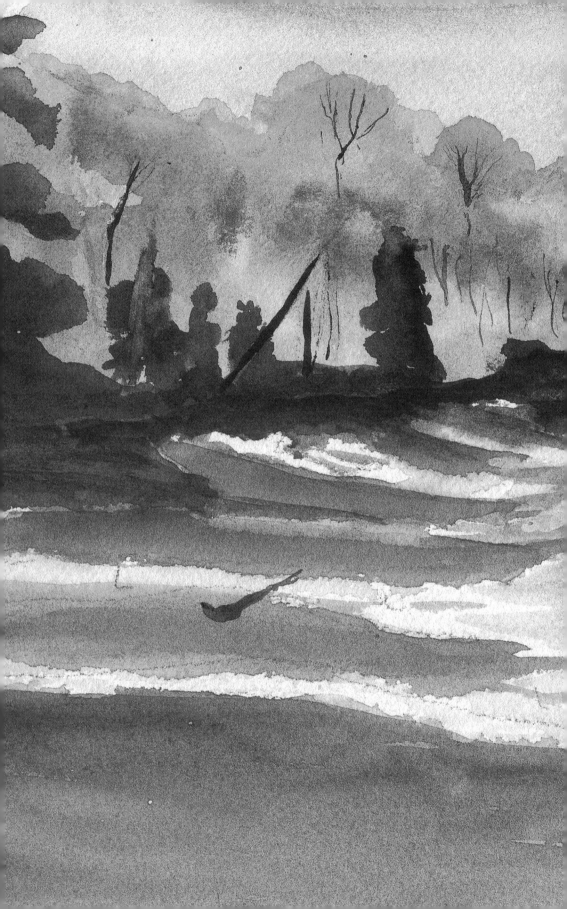

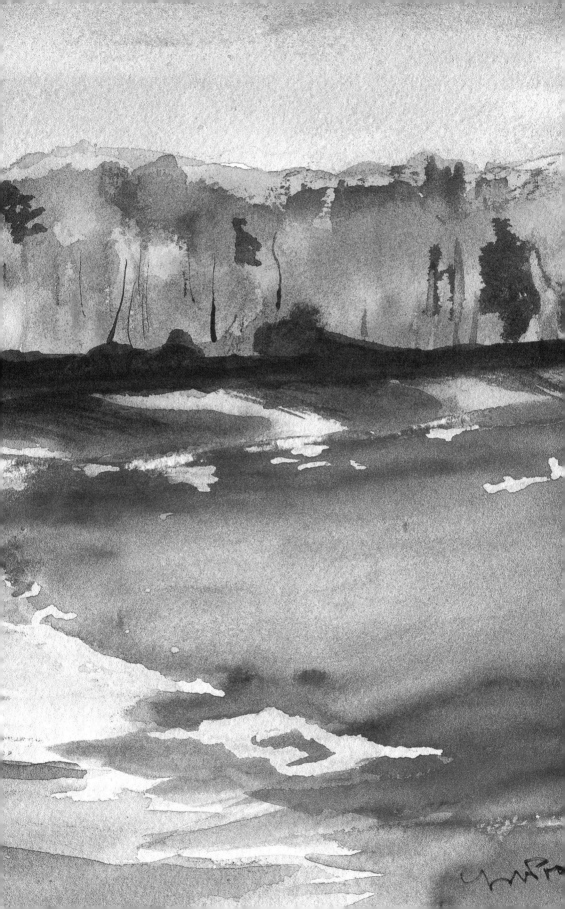

chapter twenty
the leading causes of life

...

There were 15 or so people on the conference call as the Atlanta-based Interfaith Health Program checked in with the teams it had trained to enhance healing and bring about change. A few weeks before my first stroke, I had trained one of those teams. It was time to check in with each other. What healings did the Milwaukee team have in mind for a city plagued by violence? Had anything changed? What story would our Montana team tell about healers separated by vast distances and scant resources? What was the story of the Pennsylvania team that wanted to find a seam of hope in the coal fields of despair?

Each team made a searching and fearless inventory of the ills that needed to be addressed. In each case there was an implicit understanding that analysis alone would not lead to change. I had long thought that analysis might be the cardinal sin of my generation. Although it is perfectly obvious that solving a problem requires an understanding of the problem, it had not led to much actual change. My generation seemed to be far better at performing autopsies than harnessing life.

I listened to one report after another, doing my best to keep up with the conversation and trying to switch tracks as one speaker passed the phone to the next. Not seeing them in February caused me to weep; hearing them in April made me thankful once again for the connection.

In the midst of the conversation, Gary Gunderson, the IHP director, said an interesting thing. He had just returned from a meeting in Milwaukee in which the problems that city faced were defined with such stunning clarity it nearly took his breath away. Every perception of injustice was completely accurate. It was an unrelenting study of the leading causes of death in Milwaukee. "I'd like to study life," he said to the team leaders. "What are the leading causes of life? I'm thinking they might be connection, coherence, hope, blessing and agency. I think that when they are present life happens. I'd really like to study life, instead of studying death. I wonder what the study of life would reveal?"

His idea caught my curiosity and I scribbled down a few notes on a small sheet of paper. We know what the leading causes of death are. What are the leading causes of life? And so I began writing to explore the idea. It soon became clear that the causes Gary listed were indeed life-giving for individuals, organizations and churches. Michaelangelo's painting of God reaching for Adam's outstretched hand portrayed the beautiful power of connection. The creation story is a story of coherence. Out of the chaos came order, out of the darkness came light, out of emptiness came the harmony of sky, land and water. What we do as humans is to organize and find coherence in our lives. We do so among the ebbs and flows of hope. In short, the five leading causes worked. To the list I would eventually add time.

Sometimes when I sat down to write, the words appeared. But more often they did not. I would stare at the computer screen and wait, wait, and wait a bit longer for the wheels of my thought to gain traction. In my mind's eye I knew precisely what I wanted to write, but the words eluded me and I could never quite come to the point. My writing was eloquent, but obtuse.

"That's a classic symptom of frontal lobe damage," said David when we talked about it. "Patients make all kinds of promises they can't fulfill. It's not that they are dishonest, but they have lost some of the ability to follow through. They think they are the same, but they aren't. It really is par for the course."

The loss of executive function meant I had not lost the ability to write or think, but I had lost the capacity to crisply execute. When ideas were spinning without traction I would take Casey for a long walk in the Beartooth Mountains, along the frozen river banks, listening to the sound of the water, wondering what it had to say. I never quite knew if my difficulty in finding logical sequence was a result of the strokes, or if perhaps an affirmation of my authentic nature. Once, when I gave a sermon in Paraguay, the translator said that my words were so wrapped in poetry it was difficult for her to translate.

As the conference call went on, my preference for healing rather than "fixing" surfaced once again. Despite our expectations we do not do much healing in hospitals. We receive diagnoses, sometimes emergency interventions, or sometimes medications but healing itself happens somewhere else: in our families, our towns, our circle of friends, and our faith communities whatever they may be. It continues to astonish me that when we leave the hospital there are instructions for the patient but no instructions for his or her family, and nothing for the receiving community. One day at group I drew a curve on the board. Birth marked its beginning, and then it flowed into life. I marked our short, often traumatic and inevitably fantastically expensive encounters with the medical system with a few hash marks. Each of us had experienced a few days or a few weeks in the hospital, but we would not spend our lives there. Instead we were released into the wider world. It made sense to the group but it was not a facile understanding. Hospitals foster good community relations and lots of boosters, but rarely do they actually talk about healing with the receiving communities. In short, we have yet to understand what I call the "Geography of Healing."

I also realized that rehabilitation is an almost perfect centering of life's causes. Headway gathered patients, therapists, insurance companies, prayers of a congregation, the hopes of a family, all for the sake of healing. These connections gave life. But connection alone is not quite enough. It needs meaning and order as well. The files that had spilled from their folders needed to be picked up one by one, file by file, folder by folder until language felt familiar once again and new understandings or perceptions emerged. The dish of macaroni and cheese needed to be perceived not as a single step but as a unified set of sequences that if I could just follow directions might yield a supper. The second stroke that replaced speech with gibberish also made the importance of coherence became unforgettably clear.

And so it was with agency. Rehabilitation is not a passive experience. It does not happen "to" a person. We had to show up, day after day, week after week, month after month if life was to replace loss. It takes a lot of doing. Mission takes a lot of doing. A newsletter I once wrote for the denomination was called

Missionworks. To engage in mission, one must always adapt to changing circumstances. Hope also came into focus through rehabilitation. David said to us one day, "Time is on your side." I had never heard such a hopeful sentence. Ministry may have been receding; the capacity to write may have been waning; our debts may have been mounting; but time was on our side even if there were obstacles to be overcome.

When the *Billings Gazette* interviewed a neurologist who talked about the advent of new drugs that could dissolve a stroke-forming clot if administered within ten or twenty minutes, he added that there was little hope for those who could not make it to the hospital in time. His words portrayed a picture of despair. More than that they were not true. I wrote a letter to the editor that the paper soon published.

Such a comment reflects hopelessness. After all, not everyone can get to a hospital within three hours, and not all ERs know what to do when a stroke patient arrives. But rehabilitation -- speech, physical, and occupational therapy, together with the science of neuropsychology provide pathways of hope for stroke patients who must rebuild their lives. Can we recover everything that has been lost? No. But can we create new life? Yes, we often can, arduous as the process may be. Three hours, 180 minutes can destroy our lives and our livelihood. But they cannot rob us of hope.

Blessing also made its presence known. The cedar waxwings, the return of communion, saw us through when we were on the verge of losing our way. I realized we could give blessings, or we could receive blessings, but we cannot bless ourselves. Blessing, it turns out, requires the presence of others, provides a new perspective, and renews hope.

Gary had let it be known we were working on the *Leading Causes of Life* and his idea caught fire. He organized an event at Emory University and asked if I would attend. One of my rules of life is "never decline an invitation." I said yes. David and I talked it over.

"What would it entail?" he asked.

"A few meetings, speaking to a group about LCL, that's all," I said. He winced a bit. We had talked many times about the difference between reality and my impulsive but dangerous desire to engage in life as though nothing had happened.

"How will you get there?" he asked.

"I'll fly," I answered. At group that week a mother whose daughter had been hit by a car asked a question.

"She is going to fly to Denver next week, and I want to make a card for her that she can show if anything happens. What should the card say?"

It was a good question. What should such a card say? For years I carried a card in my wallet saying I was diabetic, that if I appeared disoriented I needed sugar immediately. We wondered if Headway shouldn't make producing such a card a project. Perhaps it would say she may need to rest in a quiet place if she became confused or overly tired, and that such confusion is not the result of drugs. Perhaps it would include Headway's phone number.

I had become aware that when I entered stores, clerks eyed me somewhat suspiciously, reading perhaps that I wasn't quite "there," and had some ulterior motives. The suspicion eased once we engaged in a bit of conversation, although I kept thinking my occasionally missed words gave me away. "You're weird," a friend once said to me after seeing me in a social situation over which I had no control. "I'm trying to hold on as best I can," I answered with a bit of defensive self-justification. But I appreciated his observation, because I knew it was awkwardly true. Perhaps "the Headway card would read, "I'm okay, though brain injury might make it appear otherwise. Thank you for acting, and not reacting." I am still deeply aware that I do not fit in when I enter social situations.

"Is it a non-stop flight?" David asked about the flight to Atlanta.

"Billings to Minneapolis, then Minneapolis to Atlanta, Atlanta to Minneapolis, Minneapolis to Billings," I answered.

"You know if you keep trying to do all of this one of these days you're not going to come back," he said. Life presented its tug-of-war once again. If taking care of myself means avoiding life, what's the point? Anosognosia warped my view of what I could do. One voice said, "Be careful." Another voice, aware of economic reality, and my craving for a job, said, "You must do something." Finding a balance between them is an unavoidable chapter in each TBI/stroke survivor's story.

"I think I'll be okay," I said. Besides, this gives me hope."

"Be careful," David said. "Take care," the group said, "and tell us about it when you return."

Worried about the trip Connie had called IHP to see if someone could pick me up at the Atlanta airport, and they were more than helpful. As I walked through the chaotic terminal David's words of warning came back. On all sides everyone else knew with overwhelming certainty precisely where they were going. Only I seemed to be lost, trying to find EXIT signs. More than once I asked how to get out of the building. It was such a strange question. Everyone else knew precisely where to go. I was flooded. Hook, line, and sinker, I was flooded. Finally I left the terminal, and somehow found Neils who kindly drove me to the conference. The IHP staff greeted me and gave me a name tag and a program for the day's events. Several hundred people milled about waiting for the conference. Still unsure of exactly what I would be saying, or just when my session would begin, I headed into an auditorium which had a table up front for the speakers. Assuming I was one of the speakers, I sat down at the table.

"Good morning," said the man next to me. He was one of the speakers.

"Good morning," I said.

"Who are you?" he asked.

"Larry Pray," I said.

"Nice to meet you," he said, turning back to his papers and looking down the table toward the other distinguished speakers. I suddenly realized I had no business at that table. It was for the main speakers. I sheepishly made my way to into the crowd and took a seat and couldn't help but laugh at my *faux pas*. An hour later the group broke up and drifted into small seminars. In one of them I spoke for fifteen minutes or so about some of what I had written for the *Leading Causes of Life*. My words were essentially a sharing of the life of our church that tried to harness hope, compassion, and blessing in ways that cared deeply about the lives of individuals and their time. It was simply a matter of sharing the stories that had lodged themselves in my heart. After the session we headed for a worship service in the chapel. There were two sermons on that day. The first wrapped its insight in a gentle telling of poignant stories. "My poetry is essential courteous, but not tame," wrote the poet William Stafford in his beautiful

---

12 William Stafford, *A Scripture of Leaves*, Brethren Press, Elgin, Illinois, 1989.

poem, *Contributor's Note*.[13] The words of this sermon were also courteous, but not tame.

The sermon drew to a close.

We took a break and then reassembled for the second sermon.

This preacher laced his sermon with the strident tones of righteous indignation. In no uncertain terms he decried that God's dispensation of justice had once again been perversely thwarted. The church had been complicit and complacent as God's healing had been willfully, consistently and intentionally ignored. The presence of impatient anger was overwhelming.

Brain injury dramatically changes the role of anger in our lives. In "normal life," we know how to deal with anger. Our brains are built to protect us. Take away too many of the neurons that filter anger and it turns into a virtual assault. Maintaining a sense of equanimity in the midst of a battle demands every neuron we have at our disposal. Take away the neurons and either anger has no restraint or we fail to know how to defuse a situation. Either way there is no safety. Negotiating peace is far more complicated than waging war. Defusing violence turns out to be an astonishingly complex endeavor.

The preacher had a right to be angry. It is true that poverty jeopardizes health, that the draconian choice between groceries and prescriptions is all too common. Over and over again injustice raises its ugly head. Anger is not an inappropriate response. Amos spoke of God's anger. So did Jeremiah. Even Jesus had his moments of anger. But righteous and justified as their indignation may have been, I had to slip out of the chapel and find a safe haven.

"Are you okay?" a staffer from the Interfaith Health Program asked. My face was pale, my expression one of exhaustion, my eyes connected with chaos.

"Not really," I said. "I think I'd better lay down." Fortunately there was a couch not far from the chapel. I sat down; laid down; quieted down and slowly reassembled my life.

Once again, as it had so often in the past, a hymn came to mind.

> *My life flows on in endless song; above earth's lamentation*
> *I hear the sweet, through far-off hymn*
> *that hails a new creation*

---

13 William Stafford, *A Scripture of Leaves*, Brethren Press, Elgin, Illinois, 1989.

Through all the tumult and the strive
I hear the music ringing
It finds an echo in my soul.
How can I keep from singing?

What though my joys and comforts die?
My Savior still is living.
What though the shadows gather 'round?
A new song Christ is giving.
No storm can shake my inmost calm
While to that Rock I'm clinging;
Since love commands both heaven and earth
How can I keep from singing?[14]

14 How Can I Keep from Singing, *Worship in Song, a Friend's Hymnal*, Publication of Friends General Conference, Philadelpohia, Pennsylvania, 1996.

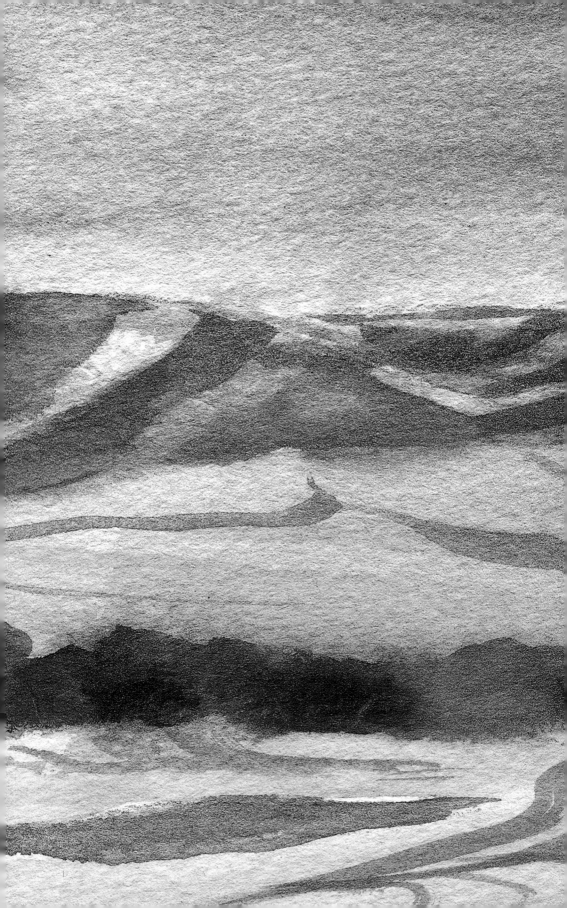

chapter twenty-one
the wider church

•••

A pastor needs a pastor.

Sometimes they fail to appear. Members of our congregation unfailingly visited us in Red Lodge, and lay members of other churches did the same, as we all held on to hope I could return. But for one reason or another my designated judicatory pastor didn't show up. Curiously I was reluctant to ask for help. When I finally did, my direct request was to no avail. Months of silence made it clear that the strokes had thrown me overboard. I had not quite fully realized the symbolic importance of a pastor in times of crisis. Perhaps we can't quite realize how important such visits are until we become parishioners. Heart-rendering movies have been made about oncologists who don't quite realize what threading the healthcare system is until they face cancer themselves.[15] Needless to say the world is full of such stories when the prince becomes a pauper, when the Word becomes flesh, when the CEO of a company disguises herself as "regular" employee and learns first-hand "what it's like." Through such experiences wisdom is gained.

Some of my disappointment may have been my own misperceptions. I somehow expected someone to speak with me not about my condition, but about the call to ministry I so deeply felt. What would happen now that the former was fading away, and the future had yet to appear? How could I discern and embrace a call that was fluid enough, and deep enough, to transcend the losses of brain injury? With whom might I have such a discussion? An unwelcome spirit of betrayal and bitterness perched on my shoulder. Try as I would to release it, it would not take flight. Instead, my outlook narrowed. It is hard to know why

---

15 One of the best is, The Doctor, starring William Hurt, and directed by Randa, Haines, 1991. Also recommended is Wit, starring Emma Thompson, and directed by Michael Nichols, 2001.

pastors do not make their calls and why such abandonment is hard to forgive. Finally, I decided I had to do something. As usual, when the student is ready a teacher appears. Bob Miller lived in Sheridan, Wyoming. We had traveled to Paraguay together, and he knew what we were up against. He was also deeply aware of Connie's struggles to make it through a day. To him, she was a person, not a "pastor's wife." Best of all, he also played the five-string banjo. I called him and asked if he had some time. Sensing it would not be a 15-minute conversation, he looked at his schedule and blocked out an entire afternoon and evening.

The drive from Red Lodge to the Big Horn Mountains is one of spectacular beauty. The country is wide and open. It isn't scenic in a calendar sort of way. It doesn't have towering mountains or waterfalls around every corner. Instead, the Crow reservation is a broad-shouldered land, its thin rivers lined with cottonwoods that that never fail to stir me, and bring to mind the verse in Psalm 1, "God is like a tree planted by the water." The horizon is miles away, as one slope fades into another. The wide expanses still reflect the way the land once appeared before its violent colonization.

I drove through Sheridan and met Bob at his church. Downstairs, in its soup kitchen volunteers were preparing meals as they did every week. We went down the steep wooden stairs to see how things were going, chatted a bit with the volunteers, before heading to his home in the small town of Big Horn. His wife, Diana, met us in the garage which, in addition to the normal array of garage implements, included her carefully tended butterflies that were just beginning to emerge from their cocoons.

The butterflies touched an enduring memory. In Minnesota, at one of our annual church meetings, three large banners framed the stage. The first was a bolt of green cloth. In its middle was a yellow circle. A brown branch, several green leaves and a voracious caterpillar chomping away at the leaves, crossed the circle. Around them an inscription read: "Live Toward the Hope in a World of Change." The second banner was made of black cloth. In its middle was a circle that framed a gray cocoon hanging from a bare branch. Once again the inscription read, "Live Toward the Hope in a World of Change." A bolt of orange cloth provided the background for the third circle in which a spectacular butterfly spread its wings. Here too the inscription read, "Live Toward the Hope in a World of Change."

The images and their encouraging message never left my imagination. Like all people, my life had its moments of voracious appetite and achievement; moments of post-stroke depression in which life seemed beyond my reach; and moments when hope's sometimes fragile wings had indeed taken flight. What I had once appreciated now swept through me again like a sermon whose every image and simple sentence made for a warm embrace. We glanced again at the butterflies, went into the house, passing by the banjo and guitar he kept on the walls, and went out on their porch, which faced the eastern horizon of the Great Plains and began to tell stories.

Bob shared the story of his pathway from general belief in the goodness of a loving God to specific belief in the abiding presence of Jesus. Like all spiritual stories, it had a theme: "I was blind, but now I see." Regardless of one's religious or spiritual belief, it is the story of everyone's life, in one way or another. There are times that specific faith is reborn as a more universal experience, and times a universal perception finds its exception and comes home to roost on a specific branch of one belief or another.

I listened. I shared how empty it felt after the strokes; how the mechanisms responsible for relationship had seemingly evaporated into thin air leaving me only with general awareness. I told stories of complaint. Why had healers never appeared? I shared stories of anguish. I kept trying to absorb everything Bob and Diana shared but came up short. It might be best, I thought, to just let it go. Surely the God who sent the cedar waxwings would continue to find a way to tap me on the shoulder and say, "I'm still here."

We spent time playing music, and then moved to their dining room table for a wonderful meal. Nothing had been "resolved," and yet everything was resolved because it was a day when the church was at work. I realized there was a difference between "my answer" and "the answer." Job's questions were never directly answered either. God answered his specific complaints with poetry so beautiful we still find it spellbinding. "Where were you, Job, when the morning stars sang together and all the heavenly angels shouted for joy?" The particulars of Job's life simply did not matter. He needed to yield to the mystery of creation before there could be resolution. The answers I sought were to be found in the depth of connection with Bob and Diana, with other clergy who had the courage to draw near the vision of cedar waxwings taking to the sky. From the beginning prayer had been announcing a presence in ways too deep for words. Prayer wasn't an event; it was the living of life and an appreciation of the sacred in life. Jacob's words told the story: "Surely God is in this place and I did not know it."

It was time to head home.

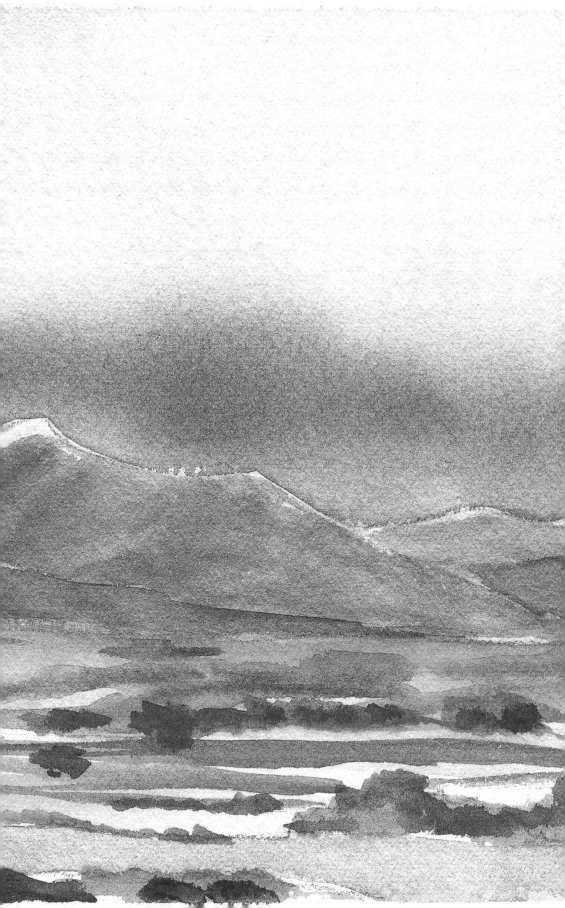

chapter twenty-two
the geography of healing

• • •

Healing has a geography.

We sought it.

We needed it.

And step by step we found it.

In November, 2005, two years after my first stroke, we could no longer deny time its consequence. The church had waited so patiently, so prayerfully, so bravely for my return. If there had been a way to turn the clock back we would have found it. Connie and I drove from Red Lodge to Big Timber for a meeting at Kirby's house. David Gumm drove all the way out to be with us and to share that despite our best intentions, I simply could not return to work. He was shocked when I implied that perhaps I could, seeing my denial as yet another sure-fire symptom of anosognosia. At the end of the meeting we set a day for the final Sunday. I wrote a letter, which I still decline to think of as a letter of resignation. It was a heartfelt chance to say thank you for showing what church can be, and for walking with us every step of the way. I could not have known that this walk lasted for years after our departure.

When the day came for the farewell service, the church was full. The presence of so many from our congregation and community was more than a man has any right to expect. I gave the sermon, which soon gave way to the litany of farewell.

"I am sorry for the times I let you down, for the things I should have done and did not do. For leadership that went astray, I am sorry." I said.

My words were echoed by those of the congregation. "We are sorry for the times we did not accept your leadership, for the things we also should have done and did not do. We also apologize."

The utter and complete mutuality of the shared words blessed us. We then affirmed each other's future, and promised to support it hook, line, and sinker.

The service ended. Connie and I drove back to Red Lodge wondering what the future held. It had become clear that staying in Red Lodge was not going to work. I simply did not have the strength, or the capacity to make a new home. It was one thing to wait for the cure that never came, and another thing to start life anew. Settling into the rhythms of a new town, takes work, care, and a measure of optimism that eluded us.

"Where do you want to go?" Connie asked me one day.

"I want to go home," I said.

"Where's home?" she asked.

"Big Timber," I said. "I want to be back where I know what the sidewalk cracks look like, where I see people I already know, where there is a relationship that doesn't need forging. I know we won't be there forever. But for now, I want to go home."

"Then let's go," she said. She checked with Kirby, who thought it could work. Everyone knew I wasn't coming back to be pastor. A new pastor would be called, and I would support him or her with all my heart and soul.

Pickup trucks with 40, the designation for Sweet Grass County, on their license plates began to arrive. In no short order we had returned home. Cassandra had an apartment she had been fixing up with the thought we might use it. We had sold our home attempting to keep up with the bills. The apartment was beautiful. Outside the back door we had a full view of the Crazy Mountains in all their majesty.

But what was there to do?

I had continued writing for the *Leading Causes of Life*. An able editor read it, and found my writing to be anything but cogent. I began splicing together the interviews with David for this book, hoping to somehow connect the strokes with a future. Writing had been both my pride and joy throughout my life. I thought I could do the book in one fell swoop, only to find it an ever-so-slow process. The stroke nemeses of sequence and impatience proved especially daunting. Perception and experience had a story to share, but its structure was elusive. We were on our own. There was nothing to be gained by another appointment with neurologists. Life itself would have to be the teacher, the reminder, and the healer.

"Do you think I had a stroke?" I'd teasingly ask Connie.

"No," she'd answer. "You had two."

"Really?"

"Really."

Not knowing what would happen on any day, many days became a matter of just waiting for something to happen.

One day a package arrived from Cheap Joe's Art Supply. It was from my mother who had embraced watercolor and music her entire life. Nearly 90, she knew the world of blocked perception might need another outlet. I opened the box. In it were paints. And paper. And brushes.

The gift said, "Express yourself."

It had been years since I had drawn or painted.

I began, timidly. A studio in the Masonic building had some extra space I could rent. The room was beautiful, full of sunlight, and a creative spirit. There was something elementally beautiful about standing before a piece of paper and, with no interruptions, with no thought of "fitting in," with no jury or judge save my own intuition, watching the intermingling of paper and paint. Watercolor is elusive, mysterious, almost etherial. It is full of change. Who would have thought red and green make for a misty grey, that a touch of red deepens a blue? Painting was a bit like rehab itself, and I never thought of it as wasting time. Instead I saw it as part of healing. The paper had to be wet, but not too wet. The colors had to mix, but only some colors did that in a beautiful way. Mostly, I was learning something. The first paintings looked like first attempts. The difference between photography and painting emerged as an important teacher. The more I tried to get a scene "right" by making it perfect, the worse the painting turned out. Accidents often led the way. I needed to find not its exactitude, but its essence, its shapes, its clean lines.

Most of all the "office" and its easel gave some sense of place, some sense of meaning, some sense of pride. I had no job, but I had a place to go, and something to do once I got there. For now, the river of healing flowed slowly through our lives blessed many times over by the fellowship and kindness of Big Timber, Montana.

In one way or another, the Geography of Healing always calls us home. It was in the spring of 2005 that my three younger brothers and I began to put together an idea. Might it be possible for the four of us, and our parents, to spend a week at Cornucopia, Wisconsin, on the south shore of Lake Superior where my Dad came of age and our children learned to walk on its sandy beaches. There would be no children, no grandchildren, no wives. It would be a return to our nuclear family. From Montana, Ohio, California and southern Wisconsin we assembled. There was something uncannily beautiful about the reunion. There we were, all six of us, at the dining room table, just as we had been before I left for college in the fall of 1965. Mom and Dad sat at both ends of the table just as they had during our youth, and the four of us took our appropriate places. At dinner we held hands and said the same grace we had always said.

> *For these and all thy gifts of love,*
> *we give thee thanks and praise.*
> *Look down our father from above,*
> *and bless us all our days.*
> *Amen.*

One day we decided to go into Cornucopia to eat at the Village Inn. They always had good fish, and we wanted to partake. We entered the restaurant, found a table for six and took our seats. A soft cascade of events began its ever-increasing flow. Around us, I could hear the voices at other tables as the waitress gave us our menus and we wondered what we'd order, knowing full well it would be fish. A series of side conversations began to arise. I began to quietly collapse, trying my very best to not let it show. There were just too many things happening at once to keep up. It mattered not that they were loving, normal, expected, and an intrinsic part of any restaurant meal. Finally the tipping point arrived.

"I'm sorry," I confessed. "I've got to collapse. I'm going out to the car, if that's okay."

They could not have been more gracious, more understanding. I went out to the car, opened the door, sat down and dozed off to sleep. They did not second-guess the decision, or come out to make sure I was okay. They gave me the dignity of trust.

It's odd in life how seemingly mundane sights and sounds turn out to be keepers. Once, many years ago, my parents and I had been talking about the sounds of childhood that had become iconic in our imaginations. Many of the memories were completely unpredictable, and had little to do with "big events."

"Surely you remember that," my brothers or parents would say.

"Actually I don't," I'd reply.

Instead it was a smell, a sound, a glimpse of light that lodged itself for safe-keeping in our lives. I shared the memory of waking up to the reassuring sound of our car as it moved from a paved road onto our gravel driveway, and my parents quiet voices in the front seat of the car as we safely returned home. None of us could have imagined that those sounds would stay with me throughout my life, signaling safety.

I do not remember my parents and brothers coming to the car in the Village Inn parking lot when they finished their meal. But I do remember them talking quietly and the sound of the gravel along the lane that leads down to the cottage. There I was, in late middle age, back home, safe in the love of family. When I was a child and heard those sounds, I did not know what the future held. And now, once again I had no idea what the future might be. I just knew that the geography of healing always leads us both home and into some kind of future that will become home.

Before we went our separate ways, there was business to attend do. Was this the time to begin talking about the estate, whatever it might be? Reason said it was. My heart said it wasn't. I resisted the conversation. Instead, I wanted us to form a circle and just "talk." A few hours before departure, we set the plastic chairs in a circle on the small lawn before the cottage. We took a small stone, and emphasized that whoever held it would speak, and that no response from the rest of us was necessary. It was a bit like a Quaker meeting. One by one, we began to share, each with a story--each with some pain, each with some hope.

Years later, I remember the authenticity of that afternoon, and how deep life-changes can be. I shared how many changes had come our way, how in the blink of an eye our lives had changed. My family's experience with disability was so very different from my brothers who had yet to go up against chronic disease. And yet we were family. We realized how quickly time was flying, and that such a reunion might not happen again.

Mostly, I was grateful that the mystery of life allowed a childhood memory to come to life once again.

chapter twenty-three
an unexpected chapter

•••

There was a church in Joliet, Montana. I knew its pastor, and one day, while we were living in Red Lodge, I decided to pay a visit. There was not a shred of irony when the choir of ten sang to a congregation half that number, and the pastor played along with his harmonica. The services were simple, safe, and graceful. Simple, in that the small congregation had only a few announcements, a sparse bulletin, and a certain joy that although the numbers didn't look good, they would not give up giving thanks for the fragile but beautiful gift of life. Safe, in that there were not too many activities for me to keep up with, and an absence of despair or ideological anger that can swamp the waters of any congregation. Graceful, in that each week they served communion. One Sunday when the pastor was away, the elder pulled out the sermon the pastor had prepared, and gently placed it aside. Instead, he stepped forward and shared how he saw Christ at work in each one of our lives. Small, it turned out, was just the right size. After our move back to Big Timber, I continued driving to Joliet for worship.

Then unexpectedly their pastor died. I shared my condolences, knowing how daunting their future might be. How could they survive with such a slim budget, ten percent of which they gave away each week? I offered to preach a few Sundays. They accepted, wanting to make sure it wouldn't be too much. They knew all about the strokes, and understood if I missed a few words, and told stories with a few unexpected and possibly incomprehensible twists and turns. I was careful to not overextend myself. I had preached once in Red Lodge. The sermon was about Zacheus who climbed a tree to see Jesus. And so, of course, I found a stepladder for the children's sermon. Kirby had said that due to frontal lobe disinhibitions, I could easily embarrass myself. I can still feel the kids and congregation looking at me up on the stepladder, asking themselves, "What are you doing up there?"

One Joliet sermon led to two, two to three, and soon we had established a rhythm of presence. They knew I wasn't the pastor, and wouldn't be there during the week, and understood it took a full day to "recover" from the drive over and the worship service. They made it clear I didn't have to attend meetings, thus avoiding the multi-tasking dynamics of committee life.

I arranged a clinic appointment with Kirby.

"What do you think about me trying to work again?" I asked. As I said the word "work," I knew it was a far cry from work. There was no sustainable salary, no health care, and no sense of full-time engagement. It was, however, a chance to spread my wings just a bit to see if I could fly, and if so, how far, and how safely.

"You know what I'm going to say," he said.

"I know."

He had been right once about the dire consequences of trying to do too much, but would that be forever true? The church paid me $100 a Sunday for preaching. The checks were deeply appreciated and helped us with the normal bills of living and the medical expenses. Mostly it gave me a sense of dignity. In October, we thought it would be a good idea to check with the insurance company to make sure it was okay for me to spread my wings just a bit. With Connie's health worsening, and her pain increasing, the thought of any change in our all-too-fragile status was to be avoided. It was important to dot every "i" and cross every "t." Their answer was stark. If I had the strength to work for an hour a week, the disability payments would stop. Period. That was it. Connie checked again. Not only could I not do it, I would have to pay back any funds the church had paid me. I would be punished for daring to try. It did not matter what our bills were, how we had lost our home. Need is never an excuse. I had been allotted a certain amount according to a certain formula, and if perchance I was able to earn a dollar I would have to pay it back. I began to feel I as though I was a thief and an enemy. In the fog of war when we signed papers right after the

.

first stroke, it turned out there was a clause saying anything earned had to be remanded to the insurance company. I felt trapped and ashamed. The only way out was to find a full-time job with benefits. I sent letters, made calls, and hoped against hope something would appear. Needless to say, nothing did.

At the grocery store one day, one of Joliet's fourth graders saw me in an aisle. I had taken my banjo to his class, told a few stories, and tried to sing a few songs with them.

"You're pastor Pray!" he said with a smile.

"I am!" I said. "That's exactly who I am!" It was a thrilling affirmation. Perhaps hope would find its way into the impasse that changed my understanding of disability. One must not only heal the mind and strengthen the body, one must enter a Herculean struggle for life with those who consider us to be an expensive problem. At its core it is a struggle for hope itself. I'd always known that hope ebbs and flows, and that when it is scarce, a smile, a hymn, a sense of irony, and stories could always help its return. This time, however, it was different. I had never felt so completely abandoned. I know I am not the only one to have fought these battles. Nor am I the only one whose misperceptions of the systems designed to sustain us are part of the problem. To live with brain injury is to live life as a vulnerable person. We resist the designation, and see in our minds who we would like to be, and perhaps even think we can be. But the truth is that we are often more vulnerable than we thought, and more confused than we realized.

The church called a meeting on a cold December morning. The table overflowed with homemade rolls, fruit, juice and coffee. Before Connie and I went downstairs, the entire congregation, all 15 or so members, met with the executive minister of the Christian Church (Disciples of Christ) to discern what could be done. She had agreed to intervene and called the insurance company to clarify what we could and could not do. When it was time for her to speak her words were exceedingly thoughtful, compassionate and careful.

"You cannot be a minister in any way, shape, or form, even if you volunteer," she said. "You can be a member of the congregation. But that is all. There could be no counseling, no committee work, no sense in which you are an unofficial pastor. You may not lead in any way. They will not allow it."

I realized in an instant that it would not and could not work. The long list of "nos" contradicted the very essence of ministry. I was also aware that I had not fully comprehended the impasse. My judgment had been lacking. My assumption that all would be well was unfounded. A letter arrived from the insurance company saying I owed them every penny the church had paid me for supply Sundays. This time new leadership in the Conference intervened on our behalf, and persuaded the denomination to send a check that I immediately signed over to the insurance company. As if to make their point, no checks were received for the next few months.

Connie's memory of these events is hauntingly stark. "As I read this, my anger comes back in waves as a deep primal force. I understood the medical reasons for avoiding counseling. But my anger runs deeper than I had even realized when a system cuts people's costs while prohibiting attempts at healing. I will never forget the looks on the faces of those dear folks as the letter was read. Shock, confusion, then anger, then the deeper anger that freezes one into silence. I've never before nor since felt such love directed to you from a singular group of solid, good people. To stand up and walk away from them was, even for me, grievous."[16]

After the meeting, we said a prayer and went on our way. Christmas Eve was just a few weeks away. This time, however, I would preach without pay, and not expecting to be paid. Christmas would not be denied. We sang the hymns, read the story that asked us to greet life once again, and lit candles. At the end of the service, nobody gave instructions. Nobody needed to. We all knew exactly what to do. Slowly, effortlessly, we began to form a circle. I lit a small candle from the altar, tilted it to my neighbor, who did the same. Soon we were all singing "Silent Night" in a room filled with light. Everything fit.

He who had never left had returned and we were there to receive the blessing of presence.

---

16 I have intentionally not named the insurance company. In the widest sense, the name does not matter. Each one of us finding our way through the collapse of our lives, will almost invariably face an opponent. It is not surprising that this opponent is financial in nature. The purpose of this book is not to pin specific blame. It is simply to share experience, with hopes that whenever you encounter snags, you will not be alone. These battles are part of the journey.

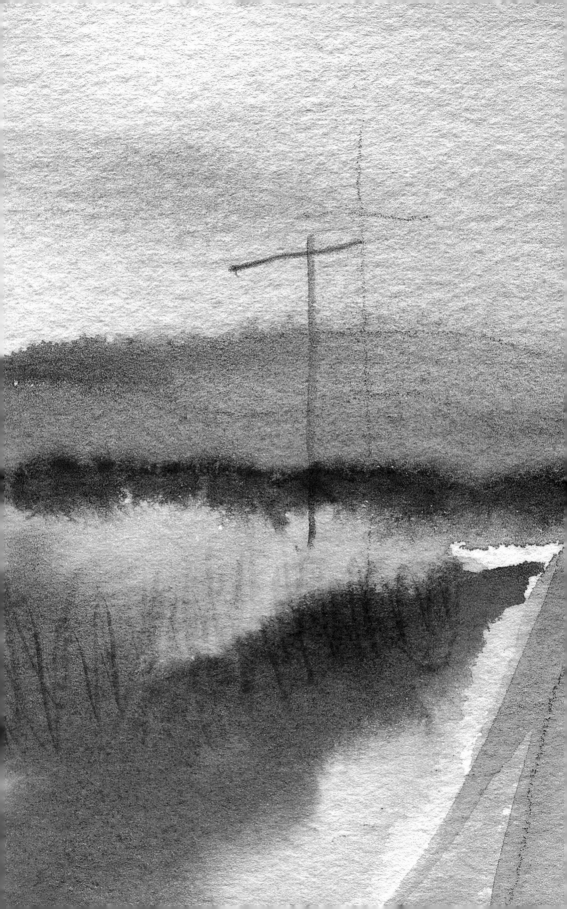

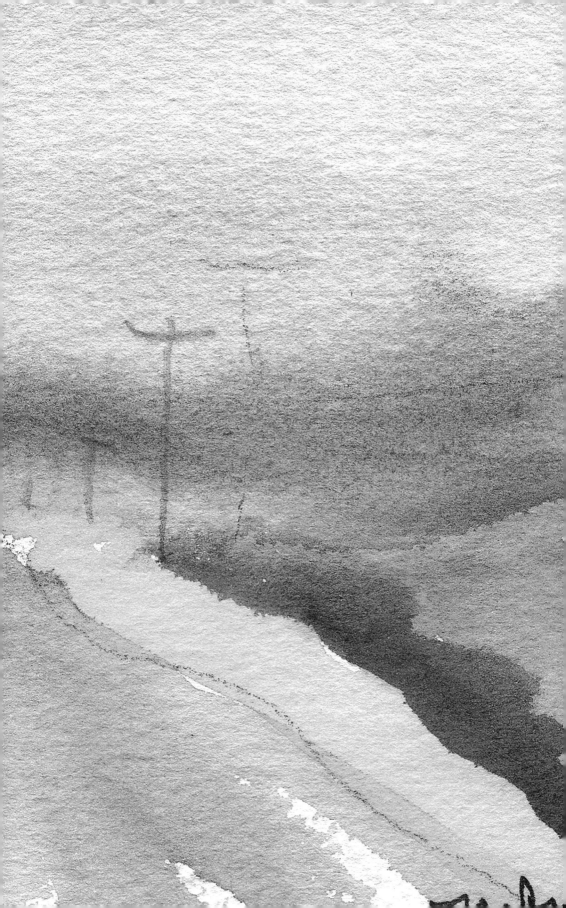

chapter twenty-four
the road calls

• • •

It had been a year since the Joliet Christmas. In the fall of 2007, the road began to call.

Something had to happen. The healings that could only come from home had run their course. Connie's situation was also worsening. A new pump that released morphine into her spine to numb the pain that had eclipsed so much of life was not working. One day I drove to the pain clinic in Billings to share that I did not think they understood or appreciated the challenge of pain she faced everyday.

"Husbands often feel that way," they said, dismissing my words. We kept hoping things would be better, but they kept getting worse. Something needed to change, and I needed to trust that instinct. If I couldn't be a pastor, might I be chaplain? Might healing be my call? Pastors live a life filled with committee meetings, but chaplains don't, or so I thought. Pastors have to multi-task. Do chaplains have to do that as well? Could my skills as a pastor lend themselves to chaplaincy? I didn't know. To be a chaplain one must enroll in Clinical Pastoral Education (CPE). It matters not how many years one has served a congregation. Chaplains must be trained in CPE.

I went online to research CPE programs.

Montana didn't have a single one.

The nearest one in Boise, Idaho, had closed.

There didn't appear to be one in Wyoming.

It looked like I'd have to leave the mountains behind. Minnesota had once been home, and so I searched its programs. I contacted the one at Fairview

Hospital in Minneapolis and asked if they would consider me. Several others I contacted never bothered to answer. I understood that. If I applied to become the world's first Type One diabetic stroke-surviving pilot, my chances of being accepted would be and should be nil. But ministry is a bit different. The idea of a wounded healer makes sense in the life the church. "He was a man of suffering and acquainted with infirmity, as one from whom others hide their faces, he was despised, and we held him of no account," Isaiah writes of the Suffering Servant that Christians tend to interpret as Christ. The voice of experience, particularly in the practice of medicine and ministry can be healing, in and of itself.

Fairview invited me to apply. Part of the essay involved writing about my experience with chaplains. I wrote about the time we were at the Mayo Clinic, and Connie had just undergone two new operations on her feet to fix the two previous ones that had not worked. A chaplain unexpectedly walked into the room and asked what was up. I briefly explained the surgery, and then added that the children had the same chronic affliction.

"I'm sorry," she said. That's all she said. But it was all she needed to say. Like the birds that somehow carried prayer into the heavens, her words somehow acknowledged God's sorrow as well. Her two words made a difference that has lingered with me all these years. That's what a chaplain can do.

Fairview accepted me.

Once again the acceptance forced a choice. There were those who said I was still too frail to risk it. Kirby had left Big Timber, so I went to Ace Walker, at the Pioneer Clinic, and talked it over with him. It was chancy, he thought, but part of life is about chance. Ace had served in Iraq as part of the Marines and his understanding of danger was anything but intellectual. There was no way to avoid risk. The only way to find out was to find out. And so, we decided to do just that. I would not be paid as a CPE trainee. Technically I would be a volunteer. But I had to try and gather myself not just for healing, but for whatever the future held. David Gumm admonished a degree of caution. He realized that my "can do it" attitude was a symptom of anosognosia. I knew his words were born of concern, compassion.

In late October I decided to visit my folks in Madison, Wisconsin, and drove the 280 miles to Havre, Montana, to catch the train. During a stop off in Minneapolis I interviewed with the CPE staff, and stayed in an apartment building right next to the nursing home where I'd be stationed. It was an interesting building. Many of its residents were one step away from the nursing home themselves, others had recently been homeless, and had been referred to the HUD building by Catholic Relief Services. Little did I know that Ebenezer Towers would become our home for the next three years and that its ever-so diverse residents would become our friends and neighbors.

We were to move the first week in January. The church in Big Timber asked if I would preach the Epiphany sermon. As so often happens, the text fit the context to a tee. Not knowing quite what they would find, the three wise men set forth on a journey following a star. We would be doing the same, leaving home in search of the possibility of a new ministry. As chance would have it, Minnesota's state motto is, L'etoile du Nord, the star of the north. As usual, on the Sunday following Christmas, we held the service downstairs in the fellowship room. There was always something anticlimactic about being in a Christmas-festooned church when Christmas has come and gone, so for years we held a stollen brunch downstairs instead. The tradition became part of our life as a congregation. I gave the sermon, thanked them for their presence and prayers, and left church for the last time.

The only thing I hadn't quite figured out was how we would get to Minneapolis. Surely I could load a U-haul myself, make the drive myself, and pay for the drive myself. But the truth was elsewhere. I hadn't quite perceived or understood how much there was to do, or how we would pay for it. Tim came home to help us pack. Emily also came home to help us pack. The moving van I thought I had arranged through the internet never arrived. Once again, the proper sequence of events eluded me. My brothers and parents had been talking about our crisis and suddenly my younger brother John arrived from Wisconsin to help us pack and drive a U-Haul truck. Connie and I arranged the car so she could lay down in the back. We began our trek out of Montana, across North Dakota, and on into Minnesota.

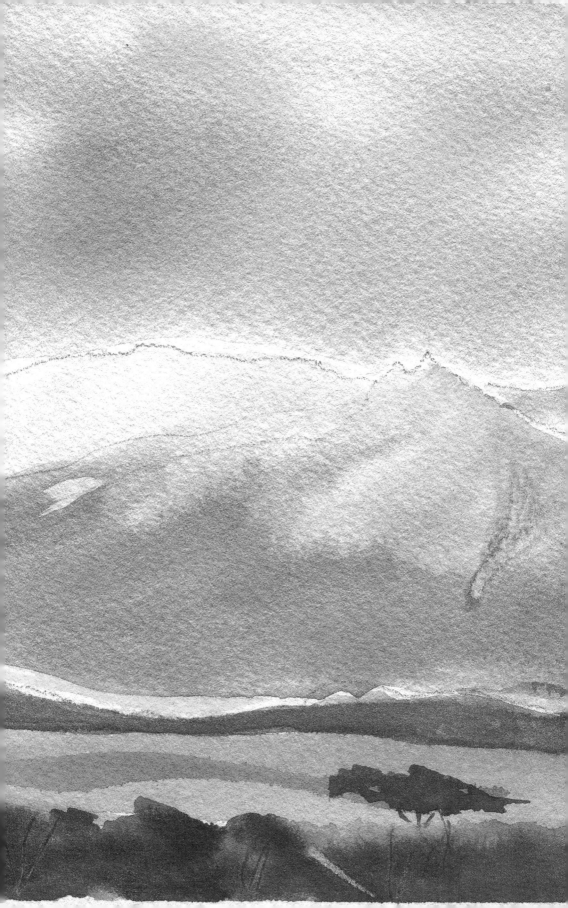

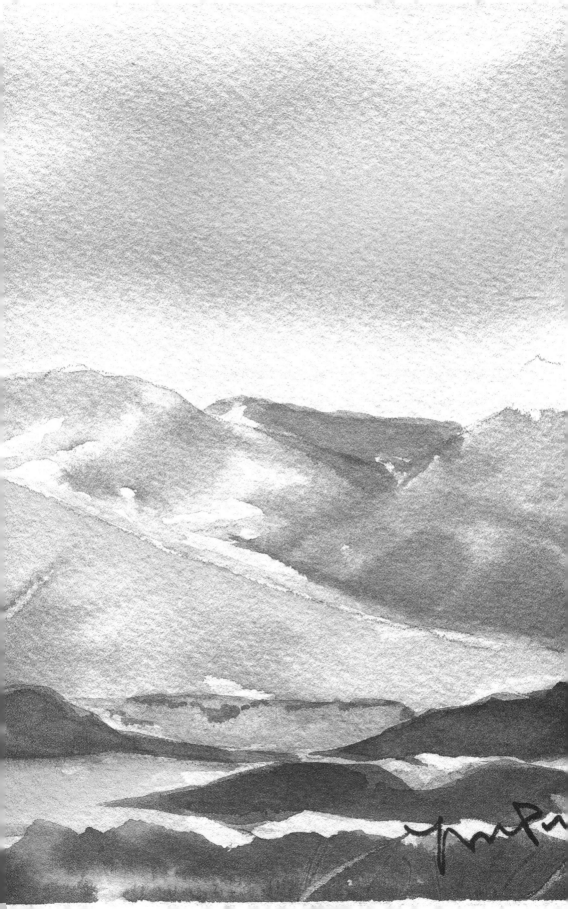

chapter twenty-five
a pastoral utrum

• • •

A strange sounding word awaited my attention.

The word is utrum. In Latin it means "whether." An utrum begins with a question. Could this be true? Yes, it could, and this is why. But on the other hand, it might not be true if you consider this, that, and some counter arguments. After sifting through the questions, and the responses, perhaps a truth would come into view. Clinical Pastoral Education, I soon found out, was an utrum in pastoral care. The questions were not intellectual. They were exercises in pastoral care.

I had been assigned to a nursing home that was just 50 feet from Ebenezer Tower. For three months I was to provide pastoral care on the dementia ward and Adult Day Care Center, while supervised by the chaplain and a CPE coordinator. Working in a nursing home was nothing new, nor were the travails of dementia. What was new was scrutiny of the six of us taking the CPE unit. We were a "group." In group we shared and dissected what happened in our exchanges with patients. We did so by writing up what are known as ver batims. In the ver batims we replayed each and every exchange in exacting detail.

What exactly did you say to the patient? came the question.

I said this, I would answer.

But why didn't you say something else?

Because.

Because why?

But what if?

What did it stir within you? What did that encounter stir within the patient? And where was God in the conversation?

Each ver batim recognized there is no such thing as a one-way conversation. There is always more going on than meets the eye, and we all have more biases than we think. Group exposed them, asked us to consider them, and attuned us to the hopes and fears of patients.

"Group" was an escalated form of rehab that pushed me to my limits. It was anything but a controlled setting, and my first few sessions were difficult. Nothing I had ever done counted. When I thought I knew something, I probably didn't. I often impulsively overstated what I had to say. It had never occurred to me in my ministry that others might not understand what I was saying, but that was indeed the case. What I thought was clear and compelling, was neither. I had never seen myself as a fighter, but under scrutiny I was fighting for every ounce of recognition and dignity I could find. As we got to know each other, I couldn't help but take the young seminarians under my wing. As that happened, I began to find my place, and even look forward to the long Wednesday afternoon sessions.

What is it like to always be thinking about justice,?" one of the CPE students asked me one day after I shared an encounter with both a patient and the "system."

"Isn't it exhausting?"

"How could we not?" I answered with a smile.

And so it went as the experienced taught the inexperienced, and we all sorted through the ministry of pastoral care.

It often took several days to recover from the group experience, and from days at the nursing home where too many things happened at once--such as gathering up residents for a chapel service or an outing. It did not surprise me that I gravitated to the non-clinical areas of the nursing home. The memory care unit did its very best to avoid the medical model. The patients exercised together, ate together, and celebrated holidays or birthdays together. The staff did not want to view their patients as "sick."

I felt an immediate connection with these men and women. I too knew what it was to lose words. I too knew what it was to know something was wrong without being able to name it. I too knew what it was to have feelings and thoughts that others could not quite put into words. They were "my people." I checked in on them whenever I had the strength which, in my estimation, was not often enough. I did the same for people at the adult day-care center, and those at a housing complex for whom I led a Bible study once a week.

I loved them all, perhaps because of our shared experience, and our mutual ability to overlook the obvious and find something else. I stood beside them as they spent hours watching snow gently cover the streets as they waited for a long-lost son to walk up those same sidewalks. I learned which ones were difficult, and made sure to call them not by their birth names, but by the names they had given themselves. I received the blessing of a serene and beautiful smile from the Alzheimer's patient who spoke but one or two sentences during the three months I knew him. In incomprehensible words, but with a depth of emotion in his eye, and a movement of his hand, he said that he wanted to talk but the words . . . the words . . . the words.

I took my banjo wherever I went.

Most of the time nobody was in the dayroom when I started playing. I did not want to "round them up" for a worship service. They knew what the music meant. Slowly, one by one, they would begin to arrive. I'd see just an inch or two of a walker make its way around the corner. Then, a minute or so later, a bit more of the walker, and finally Cathy, or Sarah, or Diane would make their way into the room. Their strength, their resolve, their desire to follow the music and see where it led, and their trust that something was going to happen, moved me almost to tears. Most of us get up in the morning and go where we want to go without much of a second thought. Not them. They gather for worship with all their strength, all their heart, and all their mind.

> Once they had assembled, I'd break into an ever so simple song.
> Over my head, over my head, I hear singing in the air.
> Over my head, I hear singing in the air.
> I say there must be a God somewhere.

They knew it.

But they couldn't follow my rhythm, and, truth be known, neither could I.

First thing I knew I wouldn't be playing Over My Head, I'd be playing Swing Low, Sweet Chariot. They would begin to laugh. I would begin to laugh. I'd start it over again, we'd all start it again, and then we'd all laugh again as the song slid to wherever songs go when they are detached from the neural network that is known as harmony and accompaniment.

Along the way, I realized my instincts as a pastor were intact. I could still laugh, tease, and care deeply for the individual lives of people. And I could still learn. One woman had been in the nursing home for years. Paralyzed, save for one hand that gave an unforgettable squeeze, she never missed a worship service. By and large, she was unable to speak. As CPE neared its end in June, 2006, I wanted to thank her for her support, and see if I could perhaps learn her story. One day I saw her in the hallway, and asked if we could spend some time together. The dining room was empty, so I wheeled her to her table and sat beside her. I asked her a few questions, and she pointed to the tablemat, and made a writing motion with her hand. I found a pen, and she began to scribble her story. It was surprising she lived after a violent attack and fall. Bit by bit the story found its way to the page.

Once there, it met with another story. A story of worship, of hope, of determination to do all that could be done, of compassion.

"Have you forgiven?" I asked. I wasn't saying she should. Nor was I implying she could. But somehow her spirit transcended what circumstance could not.

She shook her head, "No."

I was surprised. When we do not forgive our lives tend to constrict. But her's hadn't constricted. Instead, there was a generosity of spirit. We are not the sole authors and finishers of forgiveness. Of our own will we may not be able to forgive. And yet, the Spirit intervenes on our behalf.

"When we do not know how to pray, the Spirit intervenes for us with sighs too deep for words,"[17] we read. She taught me that what was true for prayer was also true for forgiveness. In the end, despite all our shortcomings, and wounds that are too terrible to understand, forgiveness works its way.

Although there is much to be said for learning in class, or learning from a book, the truth is that such learnings merely set the stage. It takes an

---

17 Romans 8:27

unexpected encounter, an accidently overheard conversation, or an utterly serendipitous event to cinch the saddle. One day I chanced to walk into the Phillips Eye Institute. A photo exhibition entitled Blind/Sight caught my eye. An Atlanta photographer had taken stunning portraits of blind men, women and children. Each was then asked to describe what he or she actually saw. One described a blanket of grey, and so the photographer created that image. Another saw streaks of light. Still another saw bright butterflies in the lower left hand sector of his vision. Photographs of the person, what the person saw, and their interviews made for a stunning exhibit.

One of the women, Anita Maxwell, had been blind since birth with no known cause. The picture of what she saw was a dark grey curtain. But her words were powerful. "I realize this, that when you're visually impaired or blind, you have to be the leader, because if you're not in the leadership role, they won't listen. I've always felt that I had to kind of live above other people and what they were doing in order to make myself known and to make myself noticed as an individual. I don't know if that is something that is good or bad, but it is one of the things that is real."

"That's it," I said. "That's it." The best way to be in a controlled situation is, of course, to control the situation, in the best sense of the word. Her perception explained why I could cherish one-on-one visits as long as my strength would allow, but something like group was beyond my capacity until I began to envision group as another congregation that I had some capacity to lead.

"Be careful," I also said to myself. "That can be an ego trip. You still have to work with others, listen to them, receive their criticisms, and be part of a team, confusing though that may be, and you must be wary of judgment, or getting stuck in your thinking." And so, the waves of the ideal and the real continued to wash ashore, recede, and wash ashore again.

In our final session of group, each of us had an opportunity to summarize our experience. I realized how many of the "rough edges" that characterized my somewhat fiery beginning had given way to a genuine appreciation and affection for those with whom I had shared the previous three months. I wrote a poem for each participant, trying to touch on their spirit, their call, and their future in ministry.

When it was my turn to speak, I read the following:

My major life events are simple to trace.

A call to church

A love of church.

A loss of church.

A call to ministry.

A love of ministry.

A hope that there is yet more to share, to learn, to say.

This cannot help but have a medical edge. In the last year I have twice lost my vision. One of my sons has had surgery for the condition that has no cure and worsens with the passage of time. My wife has had one surgery, another comes this week. To have followed the road known as CPE I have had to defy one doctor; carry another's counsel carefully, and navigate each day's encounters in ways others cannot see until, much to my dismay, fatigue takes its toll.

The stunning film, Winged Migration, tells the tale of birds who migrate from the rain forest to the Arctic, and back again. Most make it, but many do not. After breathtaking scenes of the tundra, the icy mountains of Greenland, the sweeps of Alaska, one scene is incongruous. It shows a Navy destroyer making its way through a stormy sea. An amber and a red light flash in the rain as the ship forges ahead. Suddenly a duck drops from the sky and takes refuge on the destroyer. Ah, he says, I am safe. Out of the wind, but no longer flying, he tucks his head under his wing and rests.

We do not know if he can continue the journey. Who knows where the destroyer will take him? Who knows how long it will take to gather strength? But for now, just when hope almost turned to despair, just when the flight could no longer continue, a ship appeared, and he landed. The migration continues. Thank God for the bearings that guide the duck home; thank God for the ship that appeared; and thank God for the journey. For me CPE is the ship that appeared in the night, a safe harbor that is moving along a perilous migration route I've been asked to fly.

To become a chaplain one needs not one but three CPE credits. The second credit would require the equivalent of a hospital internship--eight or more hours a day, on-call duty at night, a maze of hospital computers and codes, emergency room visits, and another round of "group." I knew in an instant I could not do that. It was also not my call.

When all is said and done, chaplaincy is short-term ministry. Chaplains work with a patient over a matter of hours or sometimes for a day or two, and then may never see him or her again. Indeed, most hospital chaplains never see the large majority of patients who enter the hospital for a day surgery and leave just a few hours later. The profession has yet to catch up with post-modern hospital care. Besides, my imagination lives somewhere else. For me, time is an essential element of ministry. I resist referring to patients as cases. If I was to be involved in a ministry of healing, I didn't want it to be bound by either time or the walls of a hospital. My passion leads me to wonder about healing "out there." I wondered why hospitals pay so little attention to churches who receive their patients upon release when it is "out there" that healing actually happens.

Towards the end of Winged Migration a market-bound boat motors its way down the Amazon River. On its deck there is a cage, and in the cage there is a beautiful parrot. Over and again the parrot tries to find a way out. The cage door has a latch, held shut with a small piece of wood. Over and again the parrot tries to unlock the latch. It seems impossible. The life the parrot once had is at an impasse. Wanting to escape as the boat continues its relentless journey, the parrot keeps trying, as though it knows precisely how to break out. Finally, it pulls the twig and the door opens. There is no one there to catch it, to punish it, to put it back in the cage. The parrot hops out and, like the cedar waxwings of Red Lodge, Montana, takes wing over a forest that welcomes its return.

I know full well that brain injury has no such latch, beautiful as it may be. But the hope of flight is as full of life as flight itself. The parrot is free, but the forest is far downstream from the one it once knew. It flies off to make a new beginning in a new place. So it is with me, and perhaps you. We live in a new landscape. For me it centers on the questions of mission that framed so much of my life, and the ministry of the United Church of Christ posed them yet again: "What good can be done? And by what means?"

I always knew the questions. But now I hear them differently as I search for the words, the images, and the expression of life.

With inner certainty I can say, "Surely God is in this place, and although I did not know it, I can now trust it."

I know the written word and painting are key to whatever the future might be.

I know a world of meaning, if not a world of self-sufficient success.

"What are you?" a woman once asked me on a plane as we flew home from Russia on the cusp of my beginning parish ministry and writing for the United Church of Christ.

"A correspondent," I answered.

"For whom?" she asked.

"Just a correspondent," I said. I realized my answer was correct, but the framework to make it sustainable wasn't in place. Nobody paid me to be a correspondent. But that's what I was. And that's what I trust ministry calls me to be.

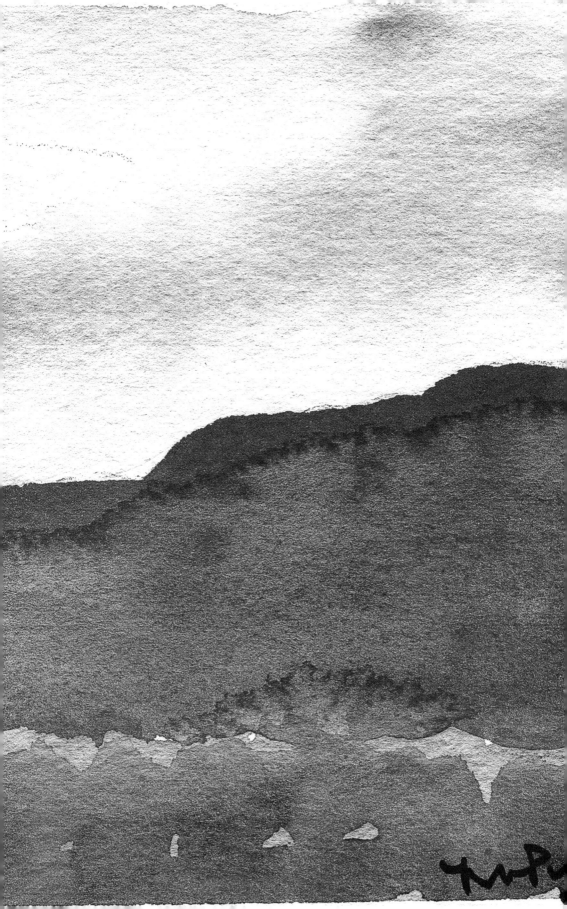

chapter twenty-six
the plateau

• • •

Once upon a time, a maple tree at the corner of Fifth and McLeod all of a sudden, dropped its blazing leaves. One by one they fell, until soon all of them had fallen. The branches were bare, a pool of blazing yellow leaves surround its suddenly stark trunk. It would be a long winter. And then, slowly at first, but then with urgency, new leaves would emerge, until it was their time to fall as well.

It was once thought that those of us with brain injuries would heal about as much as we could in a few months. Then we would plateau. Now it is commonly understood that recovery takes a good five or six years. I write these words eight years after the events of 2003. I would give most anything to find a meaningful, useful, and sustainable ending. I would like to say, "I went back to work and all was well." I would like to say, "I no longer needed disability income."

Such an ending is not yet true.

But we have continued to find a way, living in a mixture of both hope and all-too fragile circumstance. I joined a small congregation in Minneapolis that often asks us to share with each other during the service. One Sunday the question we were asked was, "Why do you come to worship when you could be somewhere else?"

"For the recovery of hope," I shared with the person beside me.

I knew after CPE what I could and could not do. A neurological follow-up test led the neurologist to say I would never be capable of working a job. If that was true, there had to be other ways to live a meaningful life. Some of that life is caring for Connie, who has had a rough go of it as her pain has increased. Her courage in hospitalizations, and her capacity to reach through the shrouds of disability to find purpose inspires me. If there ever was a family in which the blind lead the blind, we are surely it. To say this is an easy path would diminish its fierce dignity. Her path is exceedingly difficult, as is that of our children as chronic disability continues to take its toll. It takes more than two hands to count the surgeries we have experienced over the last few years, and less than one to count the successes.

We seem to be climbing not a great mountain, but a long plateau that stretches from horizon to horizon. It turns out that this plateau journey leads to springs fresh enough to slake our thirst a bit, before finding the next step. I began to work on another book, to be entitled the *Geography of Healing*. While I appreciate cures and medical fixes as much as anyone, healing is deeper, broader, and more beautiful then modern medicine sometimes understands. Those of us with chronic disease learn to accept, adapt, and find ways to live with our afflictions. Such is the very essence of our lives. It is a long process, a deeply shared process, that recognizes our inherent dignity. Good though they may be, our modern medical systems are not designed to help us live out the implications of our heart-breaking diagnoses. We go elsewhere for that--to our churches, our schools, our families, our towns. Healing has a landscape that extends over time. And so, I began interviewing doctors, hospital administrators, pastors, and friends about their lives. It tuned out that everyone had a healing story.

"I think there is a geography of healing," I'd say at the beginning of each interview.

Almost immediately, they began to share. A pediatric oncologist saw churches as places of extraordinary healing at funerals. "Who else brings us together and helps us both mourn and recover hope?" he asked. I interviewed friends in rural southwestern Minnesota who met regularly for over a year with the prisoners, and those he or she had harmed. More often than not the authentic sessions led to healing. I spoke with a physician in Memphis who shared that delivering bald babies when her hair had fallen out due to cancer was immensely healing. Some of her patients came to see her not for a physical, but to see how she was doing. Over and again, healing found its way, took its time, and celebrated new life. Its landscape wasn't a place---it was an experience.

One of our twins, Andy, called us one day, and asked me to go to the computer and log into Larrypray.com. I did. I could not believe what I saw. He had created *Praytell: The Geography of Healing*, a website for his Dad, the pastor in search of a church. Each day, I post, writing to those I do not know, sharing the perceptions, learnings, and checkmates that have come our way. I tried to have a new painting for each day's entry. Through the "blog," I practiced writing, painting, and the renewal of hope. Each day I try to exercise, work on puzzles as a continuing form of rehabilitation, and wonder what I can do to be useful to others. Although I would like to say I am not just waiting for some unexpected change, the truth is I am. But that's not to say I know what it will or can be. When we go to our doctor, she notes that I worry about Connie, and Connie worries about me. To which we both say, "touché."

From time to time I speak about the strokes. In Northfield, Minnesota, a gathering of 80 parish nurses asked if I would share my story. Each of them knew of someone in their congregation who had experienced stroke or TBI. After a nurse taught the basics of brain injury, I shared my story, sometimes breaking into laughter, sometimes tears, and sometimes passion, emphasizing how vital it is to stay with parishioners as they face the fight of their lives. A man heard the speech, and sent me two books by Temple Grandin, an autistic adult who now teaches at Harvard. Instead of trying to overcome autism, she seeks to harness its unique intelligence. He thought I was doing the same thing. At first I didn't quite understand the link. But then, I began to realize the wisdom of his words. I too needed to find ways to harness the essence of who I have become.

From time to time I am called to Methodist Hospital in Memphis, Tennessee, to expand on the blog, and to share my takes on the *Leading Causes of Life*. I have loved these trips. Methodist and Gary Gunderson are putting into place the geography of healing I hold in my heart and imagination, but cannot yet do professionally. I am stronger than I was when I first went to Atlanta. I also realize how quickly I wear out, and how when I am fatigued, I can lose the thread of a story in the blink of an eye. Nevertheless, I am among friends who ask me to be the storyteller I have always been.

In September, 2010, they showed me their new Family Care Center. In old language, it was a "waiting room" for those whose loved ones are in the Emergency Room or surgery. Such rooms have a sad legacy. They are often full of tired magazines, well-worn chairs, incessant television shows, and vending machines with the smell of stale coffee. The FCC is designed with a different purpose in mind. It is designed to care for those waiting, to connect them with their family and churches or religious community, to facilitate their conversations with doctors and nurses. They asked me if I would write something that could be given to those waiting.

"Yes," I said. "This isn't a waiting room. It's a living room. I will write for those in a living room."

To do so I drew on my times in such rooms, as I awaited the outcome of a surgery for Connie or the children. It is a place that will not allow the word "pretend." We cannot pretend everything will go well or that our lives will be the same. Change happens in a living room, just as change happens to the one on the operating table. I returned to Minneapolis, and began to write. The more I wrote, the less I liked it. I realized the last thing I'd want in such a place is a word of advice. For three months, nothing happened. Finally I threw caution to the wind, and switched to poetry and painting.

To my surprise, it worked.

Soon the poems and paintings were published, and given out at the opening of the new center. I do not have a job. But I do have a mission, one that I give away. The name of this mission is ministry. The name of this ministry is the "Recovery of Hope."

Sometimes it is in words.

Sometimes in color.

Sometimes it is elusive, sometimes lonely.

One way or another, it is alive.

"Please ask," it says. We may be brain injured, we may be disabled, we may be up against it, but we do have a life, a perception, and a hope. Let all of us then open the door and share. It may be just a plateau, but the water is sweet, and the clouds that cross the sky are unimaginably beautiful.

For the past year, we received an unexpected check each month. It came from the Montana Northern Wyoming Conference of the United Church of Christ. I did not understand why we received it. We had not asked for it. But it arrived regularly, and often made it possible to buy the life-giving medications both Connie and I need on a regular basis. I wrote back asking the Conference to thank whoever it was that provided the funds. The checks were beyond what we could ever have imagined. Pastors leave, life goes on, and former lives pass away. In April, 2011, I shared with a friend that we had been receiving these checks, but did not know their source. My friend is a member of the First Congregational Church, UCC, in Big Timber, Montana.

"Would you like to know?" he asked.

"Yes," I said.

"They're from us," he said. "They're part of the church budget."

Tears came to my eyes. Those who carried us so beautifully after the strokes, had continued to do so when we moved a thousand miles away.

As I bring these pages to a close, the maple at the corner of Fifth and McLeod finds new life once again.

So will we.

And, thanks be to God, so will you.

Minneapolis, Minnesota
April, 2011

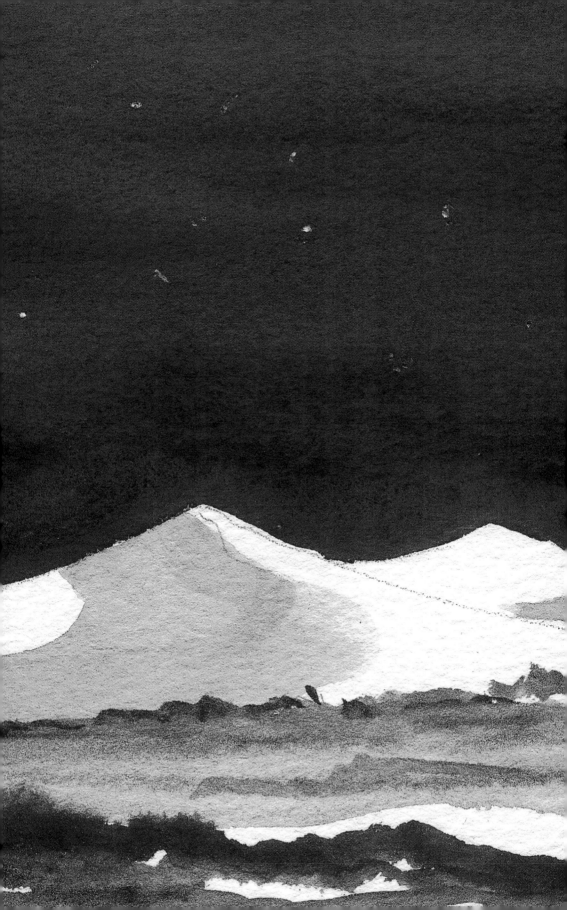

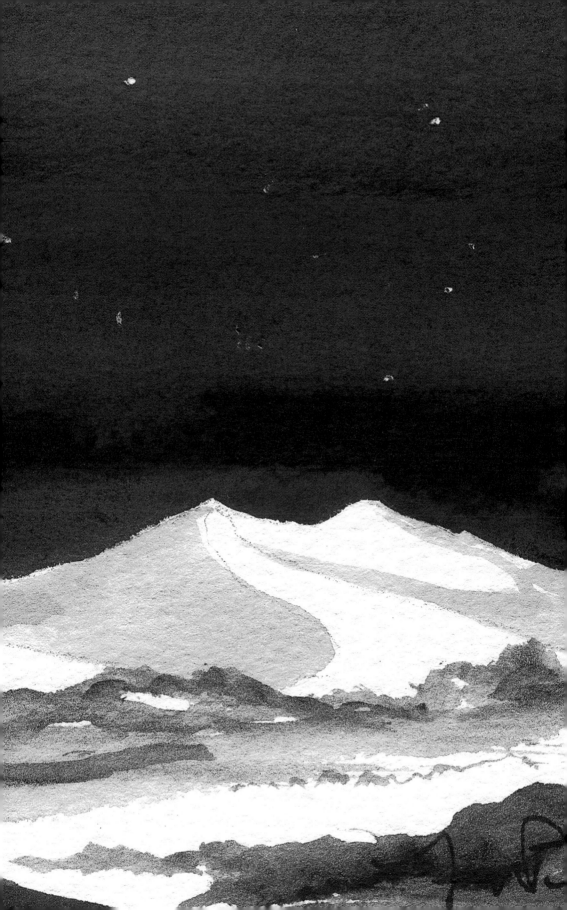

afterword
for the pastor, physician, and patient

• • •

For the Pastor

I ask you to not be afraid.

I ask you to accompany us. I ask you to join us as we try to piece together our hopes, fears, and expectations. I ask you to realize that brain injury is not an "incident." It is a life changer. I ask you to ask about these changes, and to remember that at its heart ministry of whatever faith is all about changing and mending lives. I realize this is easier said than done. It calls for some courage on your part.

We cannot speak as we once spoke. We cannot move as we once moved. We cannot understand as we once understood. But that does not mean we are not speaking. That does not mean our lives are not moving. And that does not mean we are not learning to understand God in a new way.

I ask you to not give up on us when progress is slow, when reality says, "No." I had a friend once with a severe stutter. There were so many times I wanted to finish his sentences because I impatiently didn't want to wait for the meaning to emerge. It was as though I was in a hurry, and he had to keep up at my speed.

I ask you to have the courage, and the concern, to ask us simple questions with a depth of curiosity:

"What is it like?"

"Has God changed?"

"Where is prayer for you these days?"

"Where do you fit?"

"Where now are you called?" Such a question is not only for pastors, it is a question for all of us as we search for that which is true, beautiful, and sacred. Please do not neglect such a question just because we are now disabled.

We may not know the answers. And we will need all the help you can give us to keep hope alive. We know that you cannot turn the clock back. But we do ask you to accompany us, and to forgive us when we drive you to distraction. Your visits mean more than we can or perhaps will say. Your prayers carry us and let us know that although we are detached we are not alone. These connections are life-sustaining.

Most of all, find the courage to be genuinely curious about the way the sacred appears, disappears, and appears again in our lives until, finally, everything fits. We ask you to be mindful of our condition, but to care deeply about our lives.

For the Physician

We want more than you can give.

We come to you looking for the aluminum crutch. After one of his foot surgeries, one of our twins was home waiting in a wheelchair for his bones to heal. He had to wait a month before bearing weight on his foot. In the meantime, he used a wooden crutch we had kept in the garage. One day he asked me for something unexpected.

"Dad, would you get me an aluminum crutch?" he asked.

"Oh?" I said.

"Yes, an aluminum crutch."

"Okay." Perhaps an aluminum crutch would make the difference. At the drug store the pharmacist mentioned there was virtually no difference between an aluminum and a wooden crutch. One was lighter and cost a fair amount more, but for the most part a crutch is a crutch. I knew that. So did Andy. Nevertheless we both wanted something that just might take the pain away, just might speed up the healing, just might stop the progression of his disease. We both wanted a magic bullet, knowing there was no such thing.

Our appointments with you as a physician can't help but be part of the search for a magic aluminum crutch. We know this puts a burden on you. And we know all too well that it is frustrating when you cannot heal us of all that ails us, and when the advice you give we fail to comprehend. We may not quite recognize who we are, but the stages of grief will still hold true. We will still revolt, force ourselves to overcome all we can, deny all we can, employ the magical powers of aluminum crutches, and eventually come to a new recognition of acceptance. There will certainly be times that we drive you to the point of distraction when we forget or do not understand or even resent the truth, whatever it may be. It will help us when you couch our treatment in the context of our lives. This calls for some courage on your part. It calls for an awareness of boundaries on our part, just when the boundaries of perception have been partly, or almost completely erased. It is tough sledding.

Believe in us.

Forgive us when we lose faith in your calling.

Laugh with us when you can.

Realize that the loss of our capacity to pay for an appointment means other ways of giving back must be found. Most of all, remind us that time is on our side and the tendency to compare is the enemy that gets us all into trouble.

Remind us that the injuries you can diagnose but not cure break your heart too. Such an admission will not drive us to despair. Instead, it will lead to trust. With you we will be able to look back and realize how together we found a way through the thicket of brain injury. Most of all, help us realize that although perhaps the first heaven and earth of our lives has drawn to a close, a new future is about to dawn.

On the wall of a neurologist's office I found these words:

> *The good physician knows his patients through and through--*
> *and this knowledge is dearly bought.*
> *Time, sympathy and understanding must be lavishly dispensed,*
> *but the reward is to be found in the personal bond*
> *which forms the greatest satisfaction in the practice of medicine.*
> *One of the essential qualities of the clinician is interest in humanity,*
> *for the secret of care of the patient is in caring for the patient.*

I pray that these words will frame a healing relationship with you.

For the Patient

I end by offering two five-word sentences and a three-word benediction. The first is perhaps the most important.

You have your own story. It matters. I hope the words shared here will help you find, track and shape your own story.

The second is filled with hope:

Time is on your side.

Day by day, hour by hour, something is happening. Your neurons are rearranging their priorities. They are involved in the work of creation and re-creation. Each day, even when you cannot see it, you are a new being. Each day, life is saying something to you. Life does have a language. So does God.

Know too that your fights with insurance companies, and abandonments that cut to the heart, are part of our healing. Although it feels as though they are an exception to what should be, they are the norm. The world that does not know what to make of us scarcely knows what to do with us. There is strength in a shared story. Sacred texts and stories of whatever faith, were not given to us as individuals, but as communities and congregations. It is within them that we find life.

Know too that each five-word summation has a three-word companion:

You have friends.

You may not quite know who they are, but they are there. Some of those you expect to be present will in fact be absent. No matter. Others will appear. Such is life. And this, of course, is not true just for stroke or TBI patients. It is true of everyone. Our injuries simply refocus one of life's lessons. The God you may have expected may well have disappeared. But the death of expectations does not mean the death of God. Just before this book went to press, I searched the manuscript for the word "alone." I was amazed to see how many times it appeared, reminding me that our perception of being alone may not actually be the truth. In ways we cannot always see, we are loved, appreciated, and needed. Most of all, in our singular journey we are not alone.

The words I have shared in this book have been eight years in the making. While I sensed the story, and hoped it might be useful, I did not realize what I could not have realized. I thought the first drafts were just fine. They weren't.

I thought the sequence of events made sense. It didn't. I was sure the words were not misspelled. They were. I thought what was transparent and meaningful to me would be transparent and available to others. Often it wasn't.

There was a time in my life I wrote a book every year. It took me but three months to write my first book. Surely I could do it again.

I was not aware of the losses that came my way. Slowly it began to sink in. One rejection, then another. One re-write, then another. Another re-write. Then another, each time with a bit more awareness, a bit more discipline, a bit more comprehension.

This is not a story that has a heroic happy ending. It is, perhaps, more meaningful than that. I sense what I can and cannot do, and find life to be savored, shared and cared for despite the lack of fairy-tale endings I can imagine in a flash – employment, self-sufficiency, and the capacity to earn. Comparison continues to be a foe.

"Thou shalt not covet," we read. I had never realized how key those words are to life itself. We do what we can, and must trust that like grace itself, it is sufficient. In the end, the God that disappeared returns with every tap of a keyboard, every thought of a painting, every connection with friends.

I hope that perhaps our paths will cross. In a busy restaurant, I'll probably be at a quiet table. When too many things are happening at once, I may look a bit confused. When it is time to speak, I may share a story without quite getting to the point. Perhaps the same is true for you. If we meet, know that I will wish you well, and that I treasure what we share.

"Grace, mercy, and peace" were the opening words of sermons and letters that invariably ended with these words:

And so, to you, "grace mercy, and peace."

And to you, "soft walking."

the geography of healing
travel notes

...

First Day

We were okay
until our arm,
lost its sweep,
our hand its emotion,
our voice its lilt,
our thoughts
their power to command.

The orchestra we knew so well
lost its conductor.

What's wrong? We ask.

Behind us strings
try to tune,
horns wet their whistle,
drums adjust their snares.

Still alive, we say.
Yes, but what now?
Wait and see, we sense.
And so we do.

It was day,
and then it was night.
The first day.

When Pigs Fly

Your badges said "Physical Therapy."
You asked me
to toss a heavy ball
into a trampoline
and catch the snapback.

And then you asked
me to stand on a sphere
that did its best
to turn a lean into a fall.

"Try it like this," you said.
I watched, as you gracefully
kept balance,
tossed the ball,
and caught it upon its
energetic return.

"Your turn," you said.
"When pigs fly," I said.

They flew.

What's It Like?

If we could speak
as once we spoke
words might
tell the story.

"What's it like?"
We also wonder,
as diagnoses sank in
and metallic terms–

Stroke, Traumatic Brain Injury,
Ischemic, frontal lobes,
surround us
with bewildering certainty.

In some ways it's not new.
We knew someone who
could no longer be
who she used to be.

We wonder.
Is this what it was like for her?

Who would have thought
the event that separates us
in so many ways,
also brings us together.

Shame

We've done these lessons before:
seven take away four is three.
This is how to say
pro-noun-ci-a-tion,
how to tell the time,
and lace up shoes,
and button a shirt.

We stopped thinking
about such things
a long time ago.

But now it's all new.
Don't we know how to do this?
Of course we do.
So why can't we do it?
Down deep
we are ashamed.

Despite all the assurances,
all the kindness,
all the careful therapies,
we are ashamed.

We are going to have to dig deep
to release it.
So is God
before affirmation finds its stride.

→

Rehab

"What are your goals?"

We respond to the reasonable question
with words that don't sound right,
with anger that the question
is now ours to answer.

"Give us our life back" we say.

"We can help you," they say.
"Then let's start," we say.

Our words are an ultimatum.
We must start.
We must start now.
It must work.

"Can we start tomorrow?"
"Soon."
"How long will it take?

Days? Weeks? Months? Years?

"Years."
"Yes. Here we go."

Connection

One neuron dimmed,
then another,
then yet another.

One by one
the lights
went out.

Beside them
a few remaining glimmers
sent couriers asking
if there was
anything a neighbor might do.

These sleepy cells had never
illuminated
the whole town before,
but they'd try.

Over and again,
they tried.

Soon there were new streets
illuminated by volunteers
so it is that life finds its way.

Never has creation
been as beautiful.

Could It Be True?

He had Alzheimer's.
Better said, Alzheimer's had him.

Language
no longer worked.
Neither did recognition.

"Fear not," I said, as pastors
are wont to say.

If one language leaves,
another appears.
God is with you,
and you are with God.

Trust it.
"We'll have to see,"
he said.

"Yes," I said.

And we have.

To Our Neurologists

We want you to fix us.
We know you can't,
but expect you will.

We're here
for the healings
you cannot give,
and for the assurance
you can.

We've thought with our brain,
but not much about it.
Your words are new to us:
synapses, frontal lobes,
neuropsychology,
neurotransmitters.

We prefer old words:
balance,
motion,
hope,
speech,
work,
safety and hope.

Their recovery
points the way home.

→

Graduation

Every class
has its last bell,
every month its last day.

Tomorrow
we go somewhere else,
hopefully home,
but possibly
elsewhere.

What's it like out there?
We can't know yet.
We take a deep breath,
grateful for this time here.

We
thank you.

Keep doing what you've done,
and we will too.

When we meet again
we'll have stories to tell.
No blessing is better than that.

Time

It can't always be said,
but for us
it rings true.

Time is on our side.

It blesses
our awkward learnings,
lets us fiercely deny
consequence,
forces adaptation,
refuses yesterday's scorecards,
and takes us wherever
life would have us go.

One way or another, it is on our side.

So is truth.
We are not the same.
What we've lost is lost.
But essence remains,
nesting, waiting, and
migrating to the light.

Short Term/Long Term

They want to know.
The insurance company wants to know.

Is this injury short-term or long-term?
What do the tests say?
What do we say?

Questions hang in the air.

Is there a cure?
How quick will it happen?
How much patience do we have?
How many patients do they have?

Short-term would be best.
Cheaper would be better.

We'd best find a den,
stay warm
and prepare
for the long winter
we've heard
may come our way.

To My Country

I thank you
for not shaming me.

The insurance company
wishes they could do anything
but insure.

I fight them.
They fight me.

But not you.
You were there,
to receive me
when I could not
receive myself.

I thank you
for bestowing citizenship
once again.

God gives it,
but you pay for it.

For this,
I am grateful
and owe you
a debt of
gratitude.

→

The Fit

The glove fits the hand.
In time the suit fits the body.

The silverware fits the napkin,
the fields their valley.

The shadow fits its path,
and doesn't think a thing
of finding a better fit
as the day goes by.

Age, fits its person,
as nothing else can.
Taste fits the meal
turning it into celebration.

Your hand fits my shoulder,
however briefly.

"Are you okay Dad?"
"Yes," I answer. "But it's not me."

I miss the fit.

Time itself is nothing more,
and nothing less,
than a chance
to find the fit.

To Our Regulators

Do not think
we do not know
how this works.

You must cut costs
and the numbers say
we cost too much.

Another month of therapy?
We understand
its implications better than you may imagine.

We hold nothing against you.
We too have done
what we had to do.

Forgive us,
when we fight you,
ask more of you,
and feel abandoned
by you.

Our case
is as hard as the new truths
that shape our lives.

May God bless us all.

The Unexpected

We knew the verse:
"All of creation is on tiptoe
waiting to see the sons and daughters
of God come into their own."

But we never expected
to catch it this way when prayer did not
and would not to heaven go.

The flock of cedar waxwings
alit in a single tree, beside the church door,
and stayed, quivering in the morning breeze.

When the door opened
they did not take flight.

They lingered, basking, in light.

And then,
all of a sudden,
they lifted their wings
and flew into the sky
delivering prayers deeper than words.

All creation echoes their flight:

"I'm here.
And so are you."

Ability and Capacity

How strange: to have ability
but lack capacity.

How odd to speak,
and not find the words,
to tire after a little bit of nothing,
and not much of something.

How is it sure-fired ideas
lack traction,
that a moment's victory
can't foretell the future.

How strange, this new world
that requires more courage
than strength.

We know
where the falls have always been,
and where the water has always gone.

And now?
Where did those rocks come from? How
long will the river run?

Is that the wind?
Or is that the water?

Be still. Let us pass.

→

To Our Teachers

You remind us
how to take a step,
to speak a word,
to find our voice,
and how to defy the odds.

We can be difficult.
But time after time,
you receive us,
encourage us,
asking us to do just a bit more
than we think we can,
and a bit less than the impossible.

With you
we find traction.

There is a word for this:

We call it love.

Carry On

Some heard it first
standing at attention,
waiting for release
from the order
of the moment.

"Carry on," came the order.
Life itself knew what to do.

I first heard it
from an elder,
twice my age.

"Carry on," she said.
We had done
all that could be done.
Nothing done
could be undone.
There were but two words
needed to bless
whatever came next.

"Carry on," she said.

Healing itself
did just that.

So did I.
And so will you.

For You

When we meet,
no translation is necessary.

No explanation
needed.

Your life changed.
So did mine.

Here we are,
to share a story
in search of the appropriate word.

My story,
your story,
our story,
somehow
points the way.

May
the blessings of God
be many for you,
and, along the way,
I'll take some too.

acknowledgments

...

It is said that memory and truth are cousins, but not twins.

And so it is with the events related in this book. I have written about those events I remember, knowing that Connie would have a quite different perception. Some of the events were over my head. I didn't realize or comprehend how many efforts there were, just how it was I reacted or failed to react, or what the whole story might be. The sequence of events shared in this book is based on memory and, wherever possible, notes, and keepsakes from that chapter of our lives. In the final editing of the book, the sequence of events turned out to need a great deal of revision. It makes me realize that for much of the time, I did not understand, or realize what was happening. For oversights, slights, or misunderstandings, I apologize.

I give great and glad thanks to the First Congregational Church in Big Timber, Montana, whose loving presence will always be part of my life. It is their presence and that of my family that allowed for life. What is true of them is also true of the First Congregational Church in Grand Marais, Minnesota, and the First Congregational Church in Montevideo, Minnesota, where I first learned the depth of love and care that signifies the life of a congregation.

I am grateful for the many friends who did not give up on our lives. Their notes, their calls, their patience were and are blessings. I think of the kids in Paraguay who sent an e-mail wishing for healing right after the stroke, of the team in Memphis that patiently waited for the gift of insight as I struggled to write about life. I think of the friends who somehow "kept track" of us when the news we shared was daunting in so very many ways, and those who read early drafts of the book and encouraged its completion: Ted Erickson, Teresa Cutts and Gary Gunderson at Methodist Healthcare in Memphis, Tennessee, and the noted Norwegian neurologist, Tor Haugstad, Paul Nockleby, Jim Struve, MD, Lisa Alexia, and Susan Slack, my editor at Ruder Finn Press.

And, most of all, I thank Connie, Tim, Ben, Andy and Emily for the depth of their presence and love. The courage with which they face their lives is a source of unwavering inspiration. The words shared in this book would not be possible without them.

As I waited for something to happen with the book, I shared the manuscript with my parents, Lloyd and Carrel Pray. One evening the phone rang. "Larry," my mother said. "We've been reading your book." I could tell she had been fighting back tears. They understood the yellow leaves dropping from the tree at the corner of Fifth Street and McLeod. I shared I wasn't sure the book would live.

"For goodness sake, don't give up on it," said my Dad.

The encouragement he gave on the eve of his 90th birthday is a lasting gift that will stay with me as long as I live.

Special thanks also to David Gumm, and the staff at Headway at St. Vincent Healthcare in Billings, Montana, and to Kirby Peden, MD, and the Pioneer Medical Center in Big Timber, Montana, for their extraordinary care. Ten percent of the proceeds from this book are designated to help brain-injured patients and others facing a medical crisis receive the care they need.

And I am thankful to you, the reader, who has taken the time to find your own story in the midst of mine.